AF175388

Dr Bodo Koehler, MD

The Basics of Life

Metabolism and Nutrition

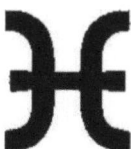

Guide to Life-supporting Medicine

Reprints or reproductions, including excerpts,
require the written consent of the author.

2nd edition 2026 (corresponds to the 5th edition in German)

ISBN: 978-3-7557-2406-3

© 2026 Bodo Koehler
Publisher:
BoD · Books on Demand GmbH, Überseering 33, 22297 Hamburg, bod@bod.de
Print: Libri Plureos GmbH, Friedensallee 273, 22763 Hamburg

The work including all its parts is protected by copyright. Any use outside the narrow limits of copyright law without the consent of the author is inadmissible and liable to prosecution. This applies in particular to reproductions, microfilming and transfer to electronic data carriers.

All rights reserved by the author Dr Bodo Koehler, MD
Cover photo by Alexander Hofner, D-Gauting

Dedication

The present book would not have come about if two great scientists had not filled this designation with what it actually means. They had the perseverance to thoroughly research the truth about our being and the courage to bring their findings to the public against all the opposition of their time. This has not remained without traces. Prof Dr Dr Juergen Schole died in 2000 of an illness that revealed the anger and hostility he had suffered. He was no longer able to reap the fruits of his labour.

Dr J. Budwig lived in seclusion until old age. She owed her robustness to the application of her scientific findings to herself, for she too had to stand her ground against adversaries and was overrun with a multitude of lawsuits, all of which, however, she won.

Both persons distinguished themselves by pursuing their path incorruptibly and straightforwardly, which is unfortunately no longer a matter of course in our time. The knowledge they acquired has already helped many people, and it is to be hoped that it will spread more and more for the benefit of all. These pioneers deserve special thanks.

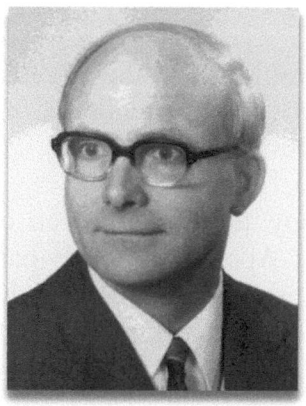
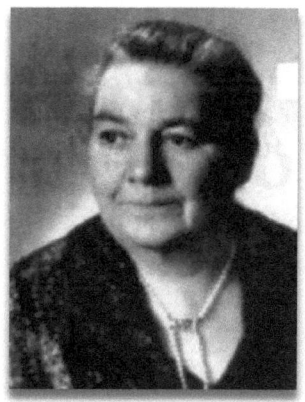

I would like to take this opportunity to thank all those friends and colleagues who inspired me at the seminars with their questions and suggestions for new thoughts and thus gave the book a special character.

Special thanks go to my wife Helga, for her patience with my work, her perseverance in proofreading and for her helpful suggestions on the chapter on nutrition.

Preface to the 1st edition

Anyone who follows the constant increase in chronic diseases over the years and looks at the emergence of more and more new unsolvable problems must at some point have doubts about the competence of our science. In medicine, I have not been able to shake off the suspicion for years that the basic approach to looking at functional processes in the organism must be wrong.

It was all the more astonishing for me when, almost a decade ago, I came across the scientific work of Prof J. Schole, who had devoted himself heart and soul to metabolic research, so that he had recognised quite different connections from the official doctrine. This was not speculation, an unproven theory, but experimentally proven research results. On top of that, they were so plausible and logical that I immediately put the new knowledge into practice. It worked straight away. It turned out that all functional processes in the organism have to be seen from the aspect of metabolic regulation in a completely different way than we are used to in order to understand them correctly. This resulted in an enormous benefit for the treatment of chronically ill patients, but also for nutritional recommendations.

A short time later, I have developed a measuring and therapy device based on these principles, which has proven its worth to hundreds of therapists over the years. Daily practice had thus confirmed the theory.

Despite all this, there were always therapy failures, or even only short-lasting successes, which was unsatisfactory. Apparently, many patients were not able to maintain the newly built up reserves, or to bring their energy balance into order. One component was therefore still missing, and this was apparently at the material level.

Through the groundbreaking work of Dr J. Budwig, I came across the fat metabolism, which had been neglected in medicine, and which not only includes triglycerides, but is the basis of the energy balance, the detoxifycation function and the acids-base balance. Her research results as a physicist and chemist had already been worked out in the fifties. Today, however, they are more up-to-date than ever.

This explains chronic degenerative processes, immune deficiencies and chronic fatigue syndrome, as well as the increasingly frequent treatment failures despite exact adherence to medical rules.

The two scientists have never met. But their findings complement each other in an excellent way. The organism can only adequately regulate and adapt its metabolism if the necessary energy is available and the full amount of life information can be provided unhindered. This is made possible on the one hand by intact membranes, which consist of fatty structures. On the other hand, we need the photons of sunlight, only a small part of which comes from food. In order to be able to absorb them directly, conditions must be created in the tissue ("solar cells") that are capable of doing so. This is made possible by fat-protein compounds together with oxygen.

The consequences resulting from the (also proven) findings of Dr J. Budwig are just as comprehensive as those for metabolic regulation. I have now attempted to create a synthesis in order to show a new path for future medicine. The primary aim is to better understand life processes (what is "life" anyway?) in order to then intervene in a purely supportive way where a deficiency has occurred. This can show itself on all levels of being and should then also be treated in its correspondences everywhere.

The basic principle of this "Life-supporting Medicine" is to eliminate burdens and everything that inhibits life – in the psyche, the metabolic regulation and thus also the nutrition, as well as in the tissue itself, the matrix. This is not a passive treatment, but an active process that has to be supported by the patients on their own responsibility. An intensive interaction takes place between patient and therapist, which has an effect on both. This sets in motion developments in consciousness that represent a communal experience.

Not only that is something special, but the high effectiveness of this new method and the possibility to help even seriously ill people in an optimal way. A positive side effect is a significant reduction in costs.

Preface to the 2nd edition

The first edition of the book was presented at the constituent Congress for Life-Conforming Medicine at the end of April 2001 in Wiesbaden. A short time later I received a call from Prof Dr Max Luescher from Switzerland, who was also a speaker at the congress. He asked me if I would like to try to incorporate the basic building blocks of metabolic regulation into his cube model. Then it could be shown whether they are generally valid statements that have a primary function.

The special thing about it is that the Luescher cube is a 4-dimensional ordering system with which generally valid connections can be created and verified.

This was of course a great challenge and exciting at the same time, because it could raise Scholes' life's work to a new level. On the other hand, if it did not succeed, then the three-component theory of metabolic regulation would not be coherent and would have to be revised.

Remarkable in this context (details in chapter 4) is the fact that Prof Dr Max Luescher developed the cube model as early as 1953. The 1950s must have been particularly fruitful....

But the present time is also fruitful. No sooner had I dealt intensively with this comprehensive ordering system of life than Dr Peter Plichta (Prime number cross) once again confirmed that reality always occurs in a quadruplicity (3 + 1 - rule). This fitted exactly with the cube model. From this point of view, it was not only possible to gain significant new insights into medicine (homeopathy, orthomolecular medicine, nutrition). It also turned out that the new theories of Prof Dr Konstantin Meyl could be seamlessly inserted and thus proved to be in conformity with life and correct. This significantly broadened the scientific basis for Life-supporting Medicine and provided an incentive for future research.

Freiburg, September 2001   the author

Preface to the 3rd edition

After a 17-year break between the last edition, the question arises: What has become different, better, more innovative in the meantime?

Certainly, we can be proud of great progress in terms of technology, electronics, new diagnostic procedures, etc. We can be less proud of the development of human consciousness. There has never been so much brutality, terror and loss of human dignity as there is today. There have also never been so many chronically ill people, suffering and misery in the world. Nevertheless, the content of this book is by no means outdated, but red-hot. We can only counter hate with love; chronic inflammation can only be healed in a way that conforms to life. Therefore, apart from small improvements and additions, there is nothing to add to the content.

In the meantime, two more books have been published by BoD-Verlag, which complement the present book or serve other purposes. One is "The Guide for joy of life in the best of health", ISBN 9-783749-48711-0, which is designed to draw from the fullness of life without harming it. It deals with all the important areas of life and is meant for everyone, young and old.

The other is "The Textbook for the UNITED Life-supporting MEDICINE", ISBN 9-783750-47092-7, which has set itself the task not only of building a bridge between the two directions in medicine, but of striving for a unification at a much higher scientific level.

In this way I would like to make my contribution to the improvement of life on this planet and the expansion of consciousness.

Spring 2018   the author

Preface to the 4th edition

This edition was created in the middle of Corona times, when people in this world were driven mad by politicians. An invisible virus was described in ever new variations as a murderous killer that leads to cruelly suffocate of the sick. Vaccination with a completely new method was propagated as the only means of survival, which was thrown onto the market within a few months, completely untested. Many people had to pay for this with their lives or suffered severe side effects.

All the uncertainty and constantly rekindled fears turned people into robots who faithfully followed every order without questioning the official measures.

The purely materialistic view of orthodox medicine as opposed to nature-pathy was blatantly demonstrated here. Koch's postulate of infection showed its weaknesses now. The human being is presented as a will-less victim, helplessly exposed to any attack without resistance. The terms "immune defence" and "resistance" were simply suspended. Instead, there were new postulates that contradict all basic medical knowledge. Healthy people were supposed to be able to transmit the "deadly" virus to other, symptom-free people. The "viral load" necessary for this no longer existed from now on. In addition, positively tested people without symptoms were classified as "infected" and thus sick, thus driving up the official figures. In the same way, deceased people were handled who suffered from completely different diseases but had tested positive. And all this was done with a useless, because extremely sensitive, but non-specific PCR tests.

What happened shows the full extent of decades of manipulation and misinformation of the world population in order to push through a certain agenda. This shows how crucial authenticity is – free from any outside influence – not only for maintaining health.

Our existence on earth should be to use every opportunity to gain knowledge and experience and to serve the divine creation. This is life-supporting.

So there is much to be done, let's get on with it!

January 2022   the author

Contents

1. Introduction

We are living in an era in which our highly technological society has ever greater difficulties in coping with new unforeseen tasks such as epidemics or the like. The reason lies in the "soulless" belief in technology, which has greatly displaced ethical values. This thinking has a particularly strong impact on science, where corruption is no longer a foreign word. Freely according to the motto "Whose bread I eat, whose song I sing".

Everything seemed feasible. Yields in agriculture were increased without regard for the side effects that this entailed. But it is these "side effects" that we are now painfully experiencing (for example, the carcinogen glyphosate), because the producers of food have *not* acted in *conformity* with life.

We are experiencing something similar in medicine. Many of the problems are home-made. Symptoms are suppressed instead of treating causes. The resulting iatrogenic damage is extreme. This has also been shown with Corona. Many of the patients died from the treatment, not from Covid 19! If the curative fever is suppressed as the first measure, cortisone, HIV and malaria drugs are used in addition to antibiotics (for a viral disease!), but nothing is done to strengthen the immune system, one is no longer surprised at the death rates. Quite a few of them are also victims of the far too often used pressure respiration (in an artificial coma). This mainly affected the elderly, whose lungs were ruptured under the excess pressure.

Only a rogue would think evil of this when he looks at the costs. An occupied intensive care bed costs 5,000 euros/day. A ventilated patient, however, costs 35,000 euros...
I will come back to the harmful use of oxygen in a later chapter.

It is not only because of Corona that we have been facing the problem of an irreversible increase in the number of chronically ill people for many years, whose treatment is tearing large holes in the health insurance system.

Everyone has the feeling that something has to change. But what?

In medicine, we should go to the roots of our being, to what really constitutes LIFE. To our great astonishment, we then have to realise that our natural science is still unable to explain this phenomenon. Nor will it be able to do so in the future, because it follows Galileo's principle and only accepts what can be measured and weighed. LIFE, however, is not tangible. There are various expressions of it that we can describe. But explain?

If we really want to establish a new way of thinking in medicine, we will have to look very closely at the foundations of our being.

In the past, there has been no lack of attempts to change medicine. There have been many useful approaches. However, they could not gain widespread acceptance because they did not touch the basis of human existence.

We cannot create something new without completely questioning the old if it is based on false premises.

Therefore, a coherent concept based on the scientific foundations of the origin of life is necessary.

What, then, would constitute a significant advance for medicine? This question can only be answered by someone who has both feet on the ground and is confronted daily with the problem of having to assign the manifold symptoms of a patient to only one (!) diagnosis. In the case of so-called multimorbid patients, the way out is usually sought by writing down several diagnoses.

If we consider the human being as a unit, there can only be one disease, even if it has different faces.

We have to assume that everything in the organism is interconnected in a network, which is why the different symptoms are also causally connected. A patient only gets a certain disease because a previous damage has already occurred in another place or on another level, e.g. the psyche.

So what is absolutely necessary for a renewal of medicine?

We need a uniform classification system that covers all functional levels of the human being and at the same time reflects the high dynamics that we encounter in the organism.

An impossible undertaking? So far it seemed so. The ever-increasing fragmentation of medicine into specialised fields went in exactly the wrong direction. Disease patterns were set up, ordered according to mechanistic points of view. If we want to maintain an overview, we need a superordinate system that is oriented towards life processes. This is exactly what meta-bolic regulation offers, as it has been excellently researched and presented by Prof Dr Dr Juergen Schole.

Such a system only needs to take nature as a model. We live in a two-part, polar (not dual!) world in which "both/and" applies. Our cells are also subject to this principle. They have to take care of both regeneration (anabolic) and energy supply (catabolic). In doing so, they interact with a variety of influences. In order to be able to grasp this, the polarity must become a bi-polar consideration.

Our world is spatially recorded in 3 dimensions. Life processes with their interactions are (related to the present) 4-dimensional, without this restriction (according to Burkhard Heim) even 6-dimensional.

So if we want to create a system that conforms to life, we can orient our-selves to this and direct our perspective to the

- **Polar consideration of all life processes** (with fuzzy logic)
- **Classification of all diseases into 4 metabolic divisions**
- **Classification in a 4-dimensional model** (Luescher cube)
- **Assignment of all influences and interactions in the system**
- **Structural order of the functional units**

This allows us to make general statements about the dynamics of the system "human being" and at the same time keep an eye on the highly complex structures that are necessary for the diverse functions. In particular, the various membrane systems should be mentioned here, which are of crucial importance for transport tasks, information conduction, networking and protection, as well as for energy balance. Their structure is therefore very special and, interestingly, is formed by *fatty acids*. Destruction of these not only leads to a loss of function, but also to a lack of energy. The *degree of order* in the tissue is therefore of great importance. This can only be maintained with energy expenditure (anti-entropy factor).

It is little known that tones and sounds contribute to this in a special way, above all the human voice (cf. fundamental tone). These findings can be used therapeutically. However, this is still a completely neglected area in medicine.

Status quo

Today's medicine gives the impression of an unmanageable science whose various fields are only mastered by top-class specialists. This means that any chance of recognising overall interrelationships is lost. The result is static observations of dynamic systems, with all the associated misinterpretations.

Science thus does not *serve* medicine, but ***dominates*** it.

"Medicine itself cannot and must not be science!" F. Sauerbruch

In fact, it cannot be, although it is often presented as such. Medicine is and remains an ***art***, because the living subject, the human being, through its diversity and individuality, permanently eludes exact scientific research. This is the reason why our natural science is still unable to explain the phenomenon of "life".

However, this does not mean that no scientific research can be conducted on human beings! It only depends on the "how". With each patient, however, the doctor is challenged to constructively transform the analytically determined individual data into an individually tailored, holistic concept and to unite it into an overall picture. This is the real art of medical practice! To do this, however, it is necessary to include the right-brain-constructive way of thinking in addition to the purely left-brain-analytical way of thinking, which is unfortunately hardly ever taught in training.

These synthetic concepts already exist, but are hardly known, although they have a strict scientific background. This refers to dynamic-regulative systems in the organism, which, however, are contrary to the usually static view. However, the human being is a ***complex, information-processing system*** with a ***high dynamic order***, which points to polarities that pervade our entire existence.

Order and dynamics are opposites and are actually mutually exclusive. However, the organism manages the feat of combining both (= determined chaos). It succeeds in this with polar regulatory mechanisms. This principle can be found everywhere. Anyone who ignores it is subject from the outset to the errors that every one-sided view brings with it. That is why we find so many contradictory opinions in science and, of course, in medicine. If science really had a firm, incontrovertible foundation – as it is always pretended to have – then there should be no discussions with differing opinions, because only one truth can exist. But since analysis always produces only individual building blocks, *partial truths* emerge and connections are lost.

This also applies to study results that, seen in them, were probably carried out accurately. But only the understanding of polar laws makes it possible to make clear, accurate statements. Under this aspect, the whole of medicine suddenly becomes manageable – one could even say *simple* – and the human being with all his or her interactions becomes more comprehensible (compare four-dimensional Luescher cube).

The university curriculum teaches a lot of facts. Every student can tell you a thing or two about that. However, since the connecting superstructure is usually missing, the first-year student must first find his way through. If he gets lost in the details, he has already lost. Only in practice does it become apparent that the wholeness of being, the integration into cosmic laws, the manifold interactions to which man is exposed, his inclinations, desires and emotions are the decisive moments, but details are rather unimportant.

Since natural science is primarily concerned with closed, mechanical systems, the completely different aspects of open, living systems are neglectted. Life runs in rhythms and in correspondences. This means that every input into the open system "human being" must result in an output that is dependent on the input. If you supply your body only with the best, you can expect top performance and you will get it. Conversely, problems arise.

Unfortunately, the latter is rather the rule in our time. The demands (meritocracy) are raised higher and higher, but usually without improving the input. Exhaustion, depression and illness are often the result. "Input" should not be understood exclusively in material terms, but (above all) also in spiritual terms.

Now, however, there are an increasing number of people who eat health-consciously, exercise, take care of their inner balance – and still get sick. This is because toxic pollution in the environment has increased exponentially, from chemical toxins to electro-smog. Even in the Amazon, radiation from thousands of satellites is a problem.

Furthermore, most people are unaware of what is "right" and what is "wrong" when it comes to maintaining health. Here, too, there are many different recommendations and opinions as a result of economic interests. However, via the track of *metabolic regulation*, the whole of medicine would be linked again – naturopathy as well as orthodox medicine.

The gap between the two fields need not exist. It has arisen from a conflict of competence about the "right" medicine. However, this question should not be dealt with theoretically. Practice must show which methods are better suited to help a patient individually and optimally find his or her cure. Which method comes into question for this must be decided quite individually, but it must prove its effectiveness. And this is exactly what bioenergetic measurement of metabolic regulation can do! VEGA-STT and -SRT, ZMR 703 or the metabolism module in MORA*nova* are suitable for this. This gives us a detection method about which there is no debate.

You are probably wondering why you have never heard of it before. In the meantime, 40 years have passed since the professor of physiology Dr Dr Juergen Schole, together with the co-author, the Salzburg physician Prof Dr Wolfgang Lutz, summarised his 30 years of research results at the University of Hanover in the book "Regulatory Diseases". In it, the "Three-Component Theory" was described, which was so revolutionary that the physiology books would have had to be rewritten. But with this, the problem was actually already pre-programmed and the theory doomed to failure. Because the scientific apparatus is far too sluggish for that.

However, those who deal intensively with this new knowledge can gain valuable insights in dealing with the various clinical pictures and thus arrive at completely new insights and therapeutic options derived from them. For daily practice, this means an invaluable gain. For this reason, an attempt is now made to present the comprehensive knowledge in an easily understandable form.

The explanations are expanded by an excursus on nutrition, which should still be the basis of every treatment today, as Hippocrates had already demanded. Here, too, inconsistencies are pointed out and new paths are shown, which result from the knowledge of metabolic regulation. Above all, the necessary rhythm is included.

Without wanting to overwhelm the reader, the biochemical foundations of life are also discussed, as they were already researched 90 years ago by the chemist and physicist Dr Johanna Budwig. This provides an understanding of the structural make-up of the organism. Reference is made primarily to fat metabolism, which is the hub, both for the structure of the cells and their energy turnover, and is not generally known in this form. As at the regulatory level, regeneration or degeneration, chronic infirmity or healing are also decided here.

2. Scientific background

Science should create knowledge about what we observe in nature. The phenomena are real even if we cannot explain them. There always remains a large discrepancy between what has already been researched and what is new before us.

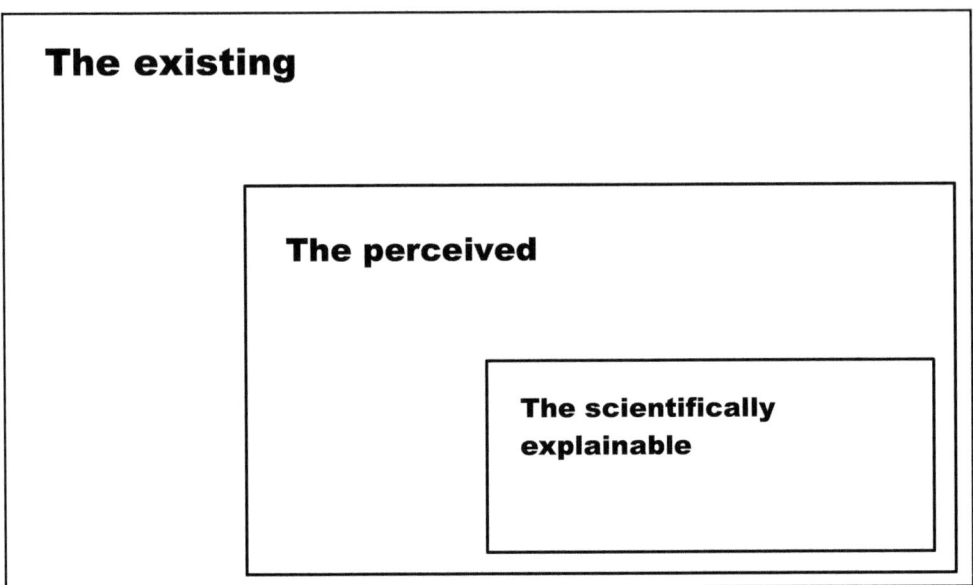

Fig. 1: The hidden part of reality

How does life come into being?
The reason why LIFE cannot be explained by our science is simple: "Life" can only be recognised by its phenomena, which can then be analytically examined and rationally justified.
That is the material aspect of being. However, this says nothing about the being itself – the living being. This is the irrational aspect. It embodies the ineffable, the mystical, the non-researchable, but the experienceable with its own, very individual cognitive value. This is constant transformation and change – the transformation of the past into a new present. The impulse for this is provided by the spirit.

Those who dare to synthesise can only guess what is really behind the phenomenon of life.

Life is the marriage of spirit and matter. Life arises where spirit can stimulate matter to meaningful action.

After these explanations, the reader will still not be able to understand life itself, but it will be easier to recognise whether certain actions or some therapies serve or harm life.

It is therefore worthwhile to take a closer look at the basics, because a very precisely examined scientific basis already exists here, on which the foundation of LIFE SUPPORTING MEDICINE can be built.

Since the connections are somewhat complicated, it serves the understand-ding to derive the different aspects one by one. For this we must begin at the source of life, the sun.

The Sun – Source of Life

Solar research is indeed the subject of scientific investigation. However, we rarely learn anything about it. I would therefore like to excerpt the views of several independent scientists who complement each other. I will start with the physicist Prof Dr Konstantin Meyl.

According to him, our hydrogen-helium sun can be understood as a huge neutrino furnace from which the earth and all life on it is fed. The neutrinos themselves come from outer space with high speed, are captured by the sun and slowed down to moderate speeds. This turns it into a pool of energetically charged, free electrons, which now have a *spin* that is very specific to the sun. This is understood to mean the angle, direction and intensity of their rotation. Electrons themselves are obviously dipoles and, according to Meyl, consist of spherical vortices, extremely curled potential vortices, with a negative centre on the outside and a positive centre on the inside. This is how they get their positionality. With the positron, it is exactly the opposite (see Fig. 2)

If positron and electron meet, they destroy each other because the direction of the vortex is opposite and they decelerate to zero - unless the centre of the vortex opens, creating a ring vortex. Then one particle could slip through the ring of the other. This can happen alternately, allowing a stable state of oscillation. At the moment of interpenetration, the charges are neutralised and something new is created – the photon.

According to this theory, photons thus represent the centre state of an oscillating system formed by ring vortices of electrons and positrons at the moment of mutual penetration.

An electron is part of a photon and can therefore dissolve back into light (just like the positron). However, it can also interact with other photons, which further excites the vibrational state energetically. As a result, electrons bound in molecules can jump to higher orbits and also leave them if they absorb further energy. They then appear as *free electrons* and are independent of the location of atoms or molecules (delocalised). However, they never deny their origin. They retain their specificity. This is also the case with the spin of the solar electrons. This has a special meaning, which I will return to later.

The French scientist, also a professor of physics, J. E. Charon, caused a sensation in the 1980s with his remarks on immortal electrons. The physicist Dr Michael Koenig takes up the subject again in his book "The Primordial Word – The Physics of God" (see bibliography). It is worth taking a deeper look at this.

The theses are presented in excerpts below:

The basic building blocks of the universe are apparently the neutrinos - tiny "forms of being" without mass, which fly through space at different speeds (including faster-than-light) and penetrate all matter.

Two neutrinos (fermions with half-integer spin) rotating around each other form a photon, a light particle (boson with integer spin). Two photons in turn combine under suitable resonance conditions (sunlight!) to form an electron. However, this does not result in a bundle of different parts, but in a highly ordered structure. This corresponds to a torus.

These black or white holes are formed by space curvature effects due to the high energy density of the photons. The difference between black and white is that black holes swallow matter irrevocably, whereas white holes transform it and spit it out again after passing through the inner funnel. Matter thus forms in one direction and dissolves back into its spiritual origin in the other ($E = m \times c^2$).

The prerequisite for this, however, is that this ring-shaped hollow body becomes charged with more and more photons that circle around in it at the speed of light. But they can also leave it again to exchange with other photons and transfer information (interaction). This raises or lowers the energy level of the electron.

In plain language, this means: The more photons have accumulated in a loving association in the electrons, the easier it is to make contact with the spirit world beyond through this dimensional gateway. For this has increased the coherence. This can also be achieved through concentration in prayer.

Electron Torus

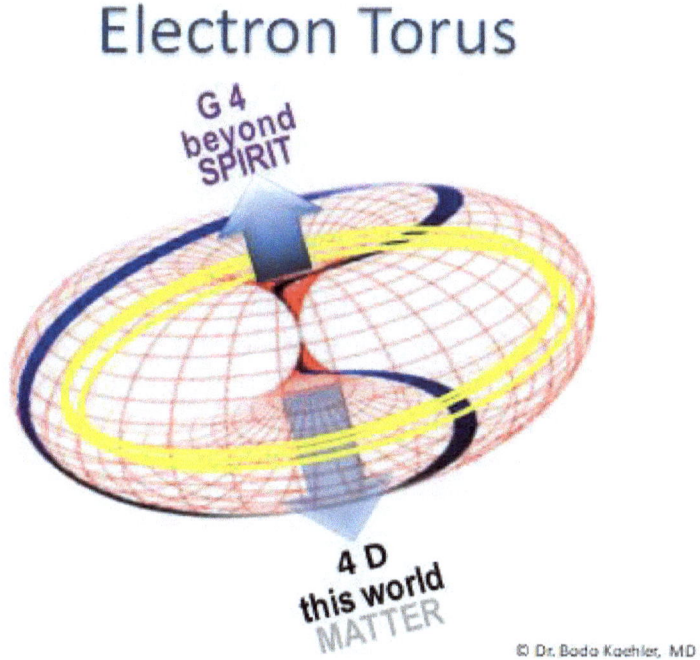

© Dr. Bodo Koehler, MD

Fig.2: The electrons charged with photons are microscopically small black (or white) holes. They are dimensional gateways between inner and outer space-time and thus establish the connection between this world and the beyong (G 4 stands for hyperspace according to Burkhard Heim).

A parallel world to this is formed by *positrons* (anti-electrons) charged with anti-photons. This anti-matter forms black holes in which matter disappears. Photons are normally directed forward into the future; anti-photons into the past and thus have a destructive effect.
The electromagnetic field of the sun (effective in electrons) is structure-forming, thus a prerequisite for auto-oxidation and cell formation (arrow pointing down in Fig. 2).

The exchange of electrons in membranes is guided by magnetic fields, as in the case of semiconductors. Due to the negative charge, electrons repel each other, but not when the information content of the stored photons differs. This makes them interesting and attractive. Only after exchanging their information, when they are thus on the same level of knowledge, do the electrons repel each other again.

So we are already dealing with consciousness processes at this level. The quantum physicist Prof David Bohm puts it this way: "The electron observes the environment as far as it reacts to a *meaning* in its surroundings. It acts in exactly the same way as people do."

Here a completely different dimension comes into play. Matter is a substrate of Spirit and therefore always reacts as a unity. Everything is related to everything else. This law works on all levels.

There are other peculiarities: Electrons create a pull of order and thus ensure a high-quality fabric. However, this is permanently disturbed by technical radiation, especially global mobile communication.

Anti-entropy factors

The photons are charged with information from their previous life experience. This makes them intelligent. They therefore possess the knowledge of the past. The further this goes back into earlier human development and the older they are, the more consciousness is stored. This makes them so-called *essence electrons*.

They can transfer their long-term experience to other electrons via resonance. This is how knowledge is always passed on. This is an act of love that can also continue in other people, creating a deep connection. This explains why couples can look more and more alike externally the longer they are connected in love.

These elementary electron-photon complexes can be understood as the smallest units of consciousness.

They are also called EIACs (Energy-Information-Exchange-Complexes), because they are responsible for the control of all metabolic processes. They thus form the scientific basis for the *bioplasm*, the often ridiculed "life energy" – the CHI.
A strong electromagnetic field keeps these complex electrons in an excited state. This is one of the many positive effects of the sun that no "vitamin" D capsule can replace.

But not only harmonious patterns are stored. All injuries are also reflected here. By exchanging the photons, however, a great deal can automatically be neutralised, namely *by superimposing positive experiences*. In this way, destiny can be transformed.

Interfering fields

However, if the incisions in life were too strong and remained unprocessed, i.e. if they far outweigh the positive, then there is a danger of repression. For this purpose, the human being unconsciously builds up a shell-shaped electromagnetic field to encapsulate this area.

Just as a histiocyte wall is erected around an inflammation on the gross level, similar mechanisms become effective on the information level. This binds energy in the form of bioplasm and leads to an undersupply of photon-carrying electrons, which means a lack of light and thus "darkening" in this tissue.

It is possible that very many people have had the experience of a *violent death* in previous lives. The anxiety associated with this can be so intense that it is one of the most intensely repressed experiences of all. A large armada of essence electrons is engaged solely in suppressing (shielding) such events. This greatly weakens vitality and can be the source of seemingly inexplicable deep-seated fears.
False dogmatic beliefs, especially in religious matters, can also bind a great deal of bioplasm, which then shows itself as an interference field. This can also affect convinced atheists.

In places with reduced bioplasm, "dents" form in the aura, which can be used diagnostically, but also therapeutically, e.g. with the balancing therapy (Equalizer EQ 103).
However, if these areas remain unprocessed (as "skeletons in the cellar"), then it is very easy to understand in Fig. 2 that the mental information cannot lead to an orderly structure. When passing through the photon ring of the electron, the primordial information is negatively altered by the contaminated photons orbiting around, which can produce unnatural forms. A tumour can thus be seen as the material image of the stored psycho-trauma.

For this reason, the treatment of an interference field is much more comprehensive than just eliminating the chronic inflammation. It is the interface between psyche and material form, as the basis for possible dysfunction and thus disease – up to and including cancer!

The structure of the tissue is built up by electrons, whereby the form is given by the stored life information (experience!) in the photons circling in it.

But the amazing thing is that *just by remembering and re-engaging* with the subject of the injury, these areas can be released from the psychological burden. Talking about it with a familiar person is automatically accompanied by an exchange of electron containing bioplasm – the unconscious transmission of experience. Often this is announced with a deep sigh of relief.

By listening well, a person can heal another person in this way completely unconsciously.

Primal fears

However, the *fear of change* plays a massive role here, because the threshold from the waking consciousness to the unconscious is controlled by fear! This is therefore a major issue for cancer patients.

The fear centre is known from neuroscience. It is located in the amygdala, which forms the front tip of the limbic system on both sides. This is significant because it provides a material substrate for symmetry in controlled action. The emotional right hemisphere of the brain should be in balance with the rational left hemisphere. If there is an asymmetry here, i.e. a preponderance of fear-producing thoughts, then cautious, considered action becomes stressful action, even panic, with greatly increased energy consumption, which can lead to catabolic derailment.

This not only increases the consumption of bioplasm, but also puts a strain on the kidneys, which are responsible for primordial confidence and calming the system. High blood pressure is therefore a seminal symptom that should not simply be suppressed with medication.

It should not go unmentioned that the new mobile phone standard 5G directly resonates with the Amygdala, which is only a few millimetres in size, due to its short wavelength and can thus trigger unconscious fears. Under fear, wrong decisions are made, which opens the door wide for any kind of manipulation.

However, the longer the double stress goes on, through deposits in the matrix on the one hand and the interference field with a lack of bioplasm on the other, the faster the nervous system degenerates in this area, resulting in a *loss of control by the brain*. Thus the further course of events is irrevocably fixed (determined). The process has now reached the full degree of autonomy that cannot be reversed by itself.

In my decades of medical practice, I have repeatedly asked myself in despair why, even after intensive therapy and a change of all stressful factors in lifestyle, turning to new tasks and a return to the joy of life, in some cases the tumour came back, often worse than at the beginning.

Here is the clear answer: The mental demands are transmitted to the tissue via the nervous and hormonal systems, and from there there is feedback to the brain. This is especially the case with inflammations. All healing processes are controlled and monitored from the brain.

However, if there is massive pre-damage on site due to deposits, loss of bioplasm with impaired oxygen uptake and utilisation, loss of information and the formation of a tissue "lump" – the tumour corresponding to the stressful psycho-theme, no therapy or other measure will be sufficient if it is not possible to re-establish the above-mentioned conditions for life in the tissue.

What is not needed is broken down. That is a law. This applies not only to muscles and bones (e.g. after a fracture), but to all organs, especially the nervous system. Shut down areas, and that is what the interference fields are, are also part of it. To make matters worse, many neurotoxic viruses are on the way that accelerate the degradation or even trigger it in the first place. These include chicken pox, for example, which can break out again as herpes zoster (shingles) in old age.
Unfortunately, vaccinations can also have this effect if they are administered to a weakened or immature immune system (babies!). Then the initial ignition is set very early.

The indispensable stimulation of the formation of new nerves (neurone-genesis) is understandably particularly difficult, but it is indispensable. Only when the organism can work again as a unit, as a whole (collective coherence), can we expect healing.

Ontogenesis

First of all, reference must be made once again to the developmental stages of the embryo and the stem cells, up to the state of full development. The reason for these stages of growth lies in the "operating instructions". It would make little sense and would only cause chaos if the entire blueprint were "played in" from the beginning. More important than the overall information is the *exact sequence* of the construction steps. Simply mixing up the sequence (while the information is otherwise complete) would cause chaos.

In a house, the roof cannot be put on before the walls have been built. If one sets priorities here, then the correct sequence seems to be even more important than the overall content, because improvisations may be permissible there. This is where the nervous system comes into play, in two ways (see later).

"Sequence" means sequence of events that must first be brought individually to their full maturity.

This regularity applies to all areas, whether it is the development of the human being from embryo to adult (phylogenesis), or individual cells (ontogenesis). Errors in the later structure and thus function can be traced back to an incorrect developmental step. This, of course, lies in the past and is therefore bound to a certain time – but also to the respective event!

Structural errors do not correspond to transformed time events!

If the "structure" is a tumour, it would be a compelling necessity to seek out the incriminating event in the past and subsequently transform it. This is not only possible, but would be the causal therapy!

However, it must always be taken into account what ground an agent hits. The state of the *whole organism* is decisive for the effect.

Life-supporting ozone layer

The light emitted by the sun then reaches the atmosphere on its way to earth and encounters the ozone layer there. This is not a passive filter as is generally assumed. Instead, the ozone intervenes directly by interacting with the photons. These are actively passed through by being absorbed by the ozone molecules (O_3) on the side facing the sun and released again on the side facing the earth. Information is exchanged through the constant absorption and reemission. The light flowing on to Earth therefore "knows" about the state of the ozone layer. The photons have been shaped by it. The special significance of this process lies in the fact that the organism thereby learns about the state of its protective shield and is enabled to induce adaptation processes in good time.

The solar spectrum has a bandwidth of 225 - 3200 nm wavelength. Of this, the range around 700 nm is best transmitted by the ozone layer (long-wave red radiation). Towards the short-wave range, the intensity decreases exponentially. At 400 nm, only half of it gets through. The ozone layer is therefore naturally programmed in such a way that only the life-promoting parts of the sunlight are sent on by it.

The remaining spectrum of sunlight is still broad enough, even if it is significantly weakened in the short-wave ranges. What is striking, however, is the strongly predominant red long-wave component.

The organism as sounding board

In our further consideration of the foundations of life, we should take a closer look at the place where the sunlight hits the organism. For the photons to have any effect at all, resonance is necessary. Certain conditions must be present for this to happen. Only then interactions can be expected. The question is only where?

We owe the groundbreaking findings on this to Dr Johanna Budwig, a physico-chemist who researched and scientifically proved the basics of energy absorption from sunlight as early as the 1950s. She came to quite astonishing findings that are of far-reaching significance for medicine. We are moving here exactly at the interface of life (cf. Fig. 3).

"Life arises at the meeting point of light and sound." Fritz Albert Popp

There are many indications from various researchers who linked the beginning of life to the reception of light. Some went one step further and added sound and still others even found mathematical laws that correspond to musical ones.

Mathematical laws

The frequencies of resonant oscillations are in integer proportions to each other, thus forming rational numbers, e.g. ½ = octave. This ratio leads to constructive interference (builds up) which can have a destructive character. This is why a military company must never cross a bridge in step. This could come into resonance and collapse.

The most stable resonance is found in the golden section. It is the furthest from integer proportions. The quotient of two neighbouring Fibonacci numbers tends towards an attractor, the golden ratio.

$$S = (\sqrt{5} + 1) / 2 = 1{,}61803398875$$

This regularity is used by the organism in a consistent manner. The Fibonacci sequence results in a natural spiral, which we find again and again in nature. The ratio of two neighbouring numbers from it, namely 21 : 34 shows the ratio of optically left-turning molecules to right-turning molecules realised in our organism. It corresponds to the quinta. If this ratio is correct, then there is a high stability, although (or better *because?*) it is an asymmetry. Life is only conceivable in asymmetry.

At the same time, it becomes clear that it can be just as harmful to take in too many dextrorotatory substances, because this disturbs the stable ratio just as much as an excess of levorotatory substances (after too much sweets). Here too, as everywhere, it depends on the dose.

Today we know from mathematics that living structures, e.g. ferns, represent so-called fractals, which can be constructed very nicely on the computer. In the meantime, a lot of research has been done on this, with the result that all life obeys these laws. The fractal (fractional) dimension D supplements the topological (integer) dimension with logarithmic values. Oscillating fractal chain systems have been discovered in neuronal networks, the hereditary systems and ecosystems, among others.
The first scientist to work with fractals was Mandelbrot. He made his apple man famous. His formula is

$$Z_{n+1} = (z_n)^2 + c \qquad\qquad z_0 = 0$$

Every bound system (like our organism) consists of bound subsystems. It generates standing waves. These connect all the components involved with each other to form a chain, which makes feedback possible, but at the same time is also responsible for quantisation (division into the smallest energy packets). The system is thus excited to natural frequencies that are fractal and have gaps. This has very special effects, which Peter Plichta already pointed out. All material appearances occur according to formula 3^4, i.e. in the sequence

$$3 - \ 9 - 27 - \ 81$$
as well as
$$6 - 18 - 54 - 162$$

The lower row comes about through doubling, thus represents the octave. As already explained above, the frequency of resolution is thus supplied at the same time. With this, every material appearance questions itself. If it is stimulated, i.e. if it receives attention, attention or physical energetic impulses, then a ***transformation*** becomes possible.

The consequence of this secret of nature is of such far-reaching importance that it is worth thinking about it for a while.

The effects on medicine can be seen immediately. If no gaps in matter would not exist, we would be a homogeneous mass with fluid transitions. Demarcation or subdivision would be difficult. On the other hand, it is precisely the presence of the gaps that makes it difficult for us to establish connections where (apparently) there are none. If we apply the ***law of four*** to symptoms of disease, e.g. cancer, then it immediately becomes clear that we are dealing with four faces, not just the tumour: cancer cells – lymph nodes – metastases – psychological correlate. All of these together constitute the cancer. If only the tumour is removed, we cannot speak of healing.

But let us now return to the electrons.

Hidden reality of electrons

As a spherical vortex, an electron has a very stable oscillation that corresponds to a quint (3 : 2). The energy of a sound quantum (phonon) depends only on its frequency ω. $E = h \times \omega / 2\pi$ as for a photon. The fundamental frequency of a vibrating logarithmic string is $2\pi / \sqrt{e}$, the angular frequency is $\omega^2 = 1 / e$.

According to quantum mechanics, we can conceive of any mass as a particle or wave (field). It is the same, just a different aspect of it. Wrong, however, would be a dualism, i.e. "either-or". Correctly, we must speak of a polarity, a "both/and". Both polar parts are mutually dependent and also control each other. No state is conceivable in which only one polar extreme exists. If one aspect comes very strongly to the fore, then the other (balancing aspect) has lost control.

The visible is always the result of a deficiency.

According to the new field theory of K. Meyl, the vibrating field was primarily present and only secondarily (through the formation of spherical vortices) did particles and thus matter come into being. According to this theory, the latter consists of stable spherical vortices, a special form of open field vortices. This view is in contrast to electrophysics, which regards the field as a consequence of the particles, but is absolutely consistent if the creative work of a higher intelligence, as postulated by quantum physics, is regarded as the origin of all BEING (cf. chapter 3 "Laws of the Universe"). The polarity then does not exist between matter particles and the field, but between the vortices and the field.

Musical laws

Overtone	Ratio	Frequency	Interval	Octave
Basic tone	1 : 1	3 Hz	Prime	Basic Octave
1. Overtone	2 : 1	6 Hz	Octave	1. Octave
2. Overtone	3 : 2	9 Hz	Quint	
3. Overtone	4 : 3	(12 Hz)	Octave	2. Octave
4. Overtone	5 : 4	(15 Hz)	Major Third	
5. Overtone	6 : 5	18 Hz	Quint	
6. Overtone	7 : 6	(21 Hz)	nat. Seventh	
7. Overtone	8 : 7	(24 Hz)		3. Octave
8. Overtone	9 : 8	27 Hz		

If we want to understand matter as wave and particle, then we should apply the laws of vibration to the wave aspect as they are given to us by music.

The quadruplicity described above can best be understood as an overtone series.
This could be continued up to 81, or 162, showing that not everything that vibrates has material reality. Reality is therefore much more comprehensive than we can perceive with our sense organs.
At this point, it must be pointed out more strongly that material structures owe their high stability only to the oscillation frequencies with which their atoms move in their spherically arranged space lattice. These are subject to the harmonic laws of music. We have Wilfried Krueger to thank for deeper insights into this (see bibliography).

For example, the formation of electrons from the oscillating state of photons is also favoured by the semitone **c-sharp**. With a natural fundamental pitch of a' = 432 Hz, this corresponds to **OM**, a universal mantra. Chanting OM goes into resonance with turquoise and strengthens the organism. Through these described connections, it now becomes clear what it can do on a material level. It thus has an anabolic effect.

OM can be understood as a bridge from light energy to matter. As a colour, OM impresses as green-blue (turquoise). This means (inner and outer) growth.

The dissolution of electrons and release of photons is promoted by the spiritual colour purple. It thus has a catabolic effect. It unites the blue with the red spectrum. Between them lies 1 octave. The colour wheel is thus not a circle but a spiral (compare Fibonacci).

According to W. Krueger, the role of the ozone layer described above is to be understood atomically harmonically in such a way that an ozone molecule (it has 3 nuclei and 3 shells) combines 12 major and 12 minor keys, i.e. 24. It has 24 protons (3 x 8) and 24 electrons in 3 shells (3 x 8). Due to the rotation of the earth, the ozone layer participates in the day-night rhythm, which means major during the day and minor at night.

The absorption of photons is strongest for ozone at 254 nm, for DNA at 258 nm and for bacteria at 280 nm. These are very short wavelengths in the UV range and are not visible to us.

Atoms and molecules are music put into form (crystallised) because they are subject to the same mathematical laws as geometry. Spatial structures and ratios have the same significance.

A Stradivarius has its unmistakable sound only because of its specific molecular composition. The vibrations of the molecules are excited from the outside and amplified into the audible range by positive interference. In this way, every material form can be perceived as a resting instrument. It only needs a push to make it sound.

Musical sounds act as external rhythm generators and immediately lead to a synchronisation of brain activity, or to a switching of the vegetative system (sympaticus > vagus), which is visible in the EEG. Higher frequencies take over via coupling processes (entrainment). This is an active process, in contrast to passive resonance.

The coupling of music into biorhythms works very well with the seconds beat (60 bars/minute), e.g. the adagio of baroque music, to increase the ability to learn.

Music is the language of matter. Photons are the language of the spirit with matter.

Tones and sounds bring the mental information into physical form. Each tone is a multiple of the original frequencies that are created when amino acids are incorporated into the protein chains. The length of the tone corresponds to the duration of the process. This knowledge is used by the

Frenchman Joel Sternberger (physicist and musician). He transfers the quantum pulsations of the molecules into audible frequencies and thus increases plant growth and resistance to pests.

The kind of vibrations we emit, we attract.

We attract things or people by "sending" a certain vibration beforehand. This comes into resonance with the same frequency and is then amplified by positive interference. This results in an effect (cf. "electron tunnel").

The effect of music on humans can be imagined in such a way that the different molecules come into resonance at different beat sequences and sound softly, whereby an intact molecule has a pure sound like a glass when it is struck lightly. On the other hand, a damaged molecule will clink.

There is not only an acoustic difference between clink and sound, which could be understood by the immune system as a signal to clear. There is also a photon emission in the form of a specific colour radiation due to the energetic excitation in intact molecules, which can be perceived as pleasant or unpleasant, stimulating or calming, depending directly on the type of music. This feeling is generated via the release of certain neurotransmitters and appeals to the soul.

The rhythm must be considered as the 2nd element of music and thus independent. The recurring sequence of tones causes resonance phenomena, which obviously have a direct influence on the nervous system, because rhythms are in the range of brain waves, but also have an influence on other biorhythms, can also overlap with other biorhythms. Homeostasis is established via rhythms (Hartmut Heine). According to Hildebrandt, information in the nervous system is encoded into rhythmic signals (iteration). Rhythms normalise physiologically between 0.00 a.m. and 4.00 a.m.

Some important biorhythms are
- **the minute basic rhythm of ATP synthesis with 0.011 Hz**
- **the heart rhythm with 1.2 Hz**
- **the respiratory rhythm with 0.3 Hz**

The ratios are interesting. The basic minute rhythm has a ratio of 1 : 108 to the heart rhythm (108 is the lunar number). The latter has a ratio of 4 : 1 to the respiratory rhythm. 4 x 108 equals 432. This is the ratio of the basic rhythm to the breathing, which is the natural fundamental of the concert pitch a' of 432 Hz. External breathing (absorption of PRANA) and ATP synthesis (through internal breathing) are thus linked via the (correctly tuned) music.

Decisive for the assessment of rhythmic behaviour is whether the rhythm is rigidly maintained or subject to fluctuations. Rigidity means loss of adaptability and contains a great potential for illness. Vitality is expressed by "wobbling" around a normal value. This fluctuation is caused by the constant absorption and re-emission of photons. Another cause is the change of location of the electron clouds (bioplasma) as the *non-fixed location relationship* (see below).

Music has sound and rhythm. It brings order into being (structure), because with it the archaic basic patterns are called up audibly.

Because classical music is played by hand, all the natural (inaudible) fluctuations of the musicians are included, which makes the music alive. Computer-generated music carries the danger of fixing the rhythms and can therefore promote illness (rigidity) (cf. techno music).

The reason for this excursion into music was to try and make clear that most of what happens "behind the scenes" (like in a play) and we only perceive a fraction of reality. But there, work is done according to a precisely defined stage plan of which we only know a few laws.
Nothing happens by chance. There is a *meaning* and an assignment for everything. It is the same with sunlight when it hits our organism. What happens here?

Intensive preparatory work is carried out in the body structures and precautions are taken to absorb as many photons as possible. Electrons are particularly capable of this, as has already been explained. These must therefore be made available in as large a number as possible as free electrons. Fig. 4 shows how our organism manages this and which mechanisms are effective.

Material prerequisites for photon resonance

The scientific findings presented in the following are based, among other things, on statements by recognised researchers and Nobel Prize winners. On the absorption of light, B. Eistert and L. Pauling on light absorption, the physicist and chemist J. Budwig and the Swedish biochemist and physician

v. Euler on the integration of fats into the living system, I. Bang on fat metabolism, H. C. F. Dessauer on quantum biology, P. Plichta and H. D. Jensen on mathematical order, A. Einstein, Rosen, Podolski on quantum physics (synchronous spin behaviour of paired particles), E. Schroedinger (anti-entropy factor), W. Pauli (resonance laws), on atomic harmonics W. Krueger, on electrodynamics Maxwell (wave equation), on spin resonance G. Schoffa, on field theory K. Meyl, on biophoton research F. A. Popp and many others.

Fats

The first prerequisite that must be created is the provision of *highly unsaturated fatty acids*. Since not everyone is versed in chemistry, first a brief explanation.

Fats are compounds of fatty acids with glycerine. Scientifically, only the glycerol ester with a naturally occurring fatty acid is considered a fat. This characterises the fat, depending on whether it is short or long chain, saturated or unsaturated. Saturated means that all C atoms (carbon) are occupied by H atoms (hydrogen). Short-chain fatty acids are easily broken down, even if they are saturated, e.g. butter.

Oils are long-chain fatty acids. They usually contain 18 C atoms (compare overtone series). Because of this and depending on the arrangement of their double bonds (cis versus trans), they are liquid. The light spectrum they absorb depends on their length. The longer the chain, the longer the wavelength. 18 C-atoms represent the optimum for the absorption of red light at 6900 Å.

Animal fats only become solid after death. The liquid form means life. Precipitation and secretion of fat indicates degeneration. Cell damage is recognised by this (e.g. lipofuscin in fatty liver).

Saturated fats cannot form compounds with the sulphhydryl groups (SH groups) of proteins and form water-soluble lipoproteids. That is why they precipitate. SH groups are components of insulin and glutathione, among others.

Oxygen

Secondly, *oxygen uptake* plays a role. The uptake and utilisation of oxygen in the organism is controlled by the *electron systems of the fatty acids* in interaction with the *sulphydryl group of the proteins*. Highly unsaturated fatty acids (especially linoleic and linolenic acids, but also mercaptoamino acids) oxidise very quickly and intensively (autoxidation) because they have a very high affinity for oxygen. They are the ones that take O_2 from the bloodstream and make it available to the cell (oxygen suction; internal respiration). A blockade of oxygen uptake due to a lack of unsaturated fatty acids means a reduction in anabolic activity and thus a stop in cell growth (lack of differentiation).

Otto Warburg had been searching for this missing link in cellular respiration for a very long time, but without finding it. He had to stop his experiments with butyric acid without results. Johanna Budwig deserves the credit for the first discovery of the role of highly unsaturated fatty acids (di-ene and tri-enes). They conduct electrons very well and are very resonant in the region of the π-electron cloud. However, besides electrons, they also transport oxygen in the blood (besides haemoglobin). Since our blood vessels are constructed like coils, the passing of electric charges leads to an induction of ring magnetic fields.

Hydrogen bonds with π-electrons

The best possibility for the supply of electrons is offered by so-called hydrogen bridges, on which *free π-electron pairs* are located. These are in resonance with each other, but this can only occur according to certain laws (W. Pauli) depending on the spin and thus the electromagnetic properties.

According to L. Pauling, the hydrogen bridge is the only way for the directed exchange of electrons in the living substrate. To achieve this, highly unsaturated fatty acids are needed (linolenic acid is very suitable), as well as protein compounds that have many sulphhydryl groups (e.g. lean curd). *Hydrogen bridges* can form between the oxygen bound to the fatty acid and the sulphhydryl group of the proteins by creating *mesomeric bonds*. Fats and proteins have thus become oxygenated *lipoproteins*. The π-electrons interact with the H^+-ions.

Highly unsaturated fatty acids act as electron donors, are therefore basic and represent an important acid buffer. At the same time, they are the most important energy carrier and indispensable for oxygen exchange. Acidosis and lack of energy indicate the absence of these essential components of our organism.

This would create the sounding board for the absorption of photons. We are here at the *interface of life*. But life is more than matter. In order to really understand what is going on here, we need to take a closer look at the dynamics. It is such a sophisticated system, largely explored in its details, that it demands the very highest respect for our Creator.

Matter is always past. Light is future. At the interface of life, the two meet and form the present.

Electron tunnel

Delocalised (free) π-electron pairs can form at the hydrogen bonds, which are called electron gas. Since electrons are constantly rotating, i.e. oscillating, a magnetic field is created around them that is perpendicular to the direction of rotation. This field forms a kind of tube, the so-called *electron tunnel*. Red light is emitted through this tube, which comes from the hydrogen atoms of the sulphydryl group.

This creates a high affinity to the long-wave red radiation of the sunlight at 6900 Å, it is literally attracted by it.

This attraction is all the greater the more double bonds with π-electrons there are in a fatty acid chain (with up to 18 carbon atoms). These must lie in the iso-electric point and be capable of delocalising the electron systems in *mesomeric bonds* (to the sulphydryl group of the proteins). This system is capable of *bipolarity* of free oxygen and activated hydrogen (which then emits red light) to then enable the life process via autoxydation with energy from sunlight.

Photon absorption

Linseed oil is 3-fold unsaturated (compared to olive oil only 1-fold) and fulfils these requirements best when mixed with lean curd. The electrons of the lipoproteids (fat-protein compounds) become charged with the photons and thus enter a higher state of excitation. However, it is crucial that they have the same spin as the sun's electrons.

This can only be understood via the well-known Einstein-Rosen-Podolski paradox. This assumes that twin particles carry out every spin change together, regardless of their position, i.e. even if they are far away from each other. The sun's electrons and those in our bodies must therefore necessarily have the same natural origin, otherwise this would not work. We are obviously children of the sun.

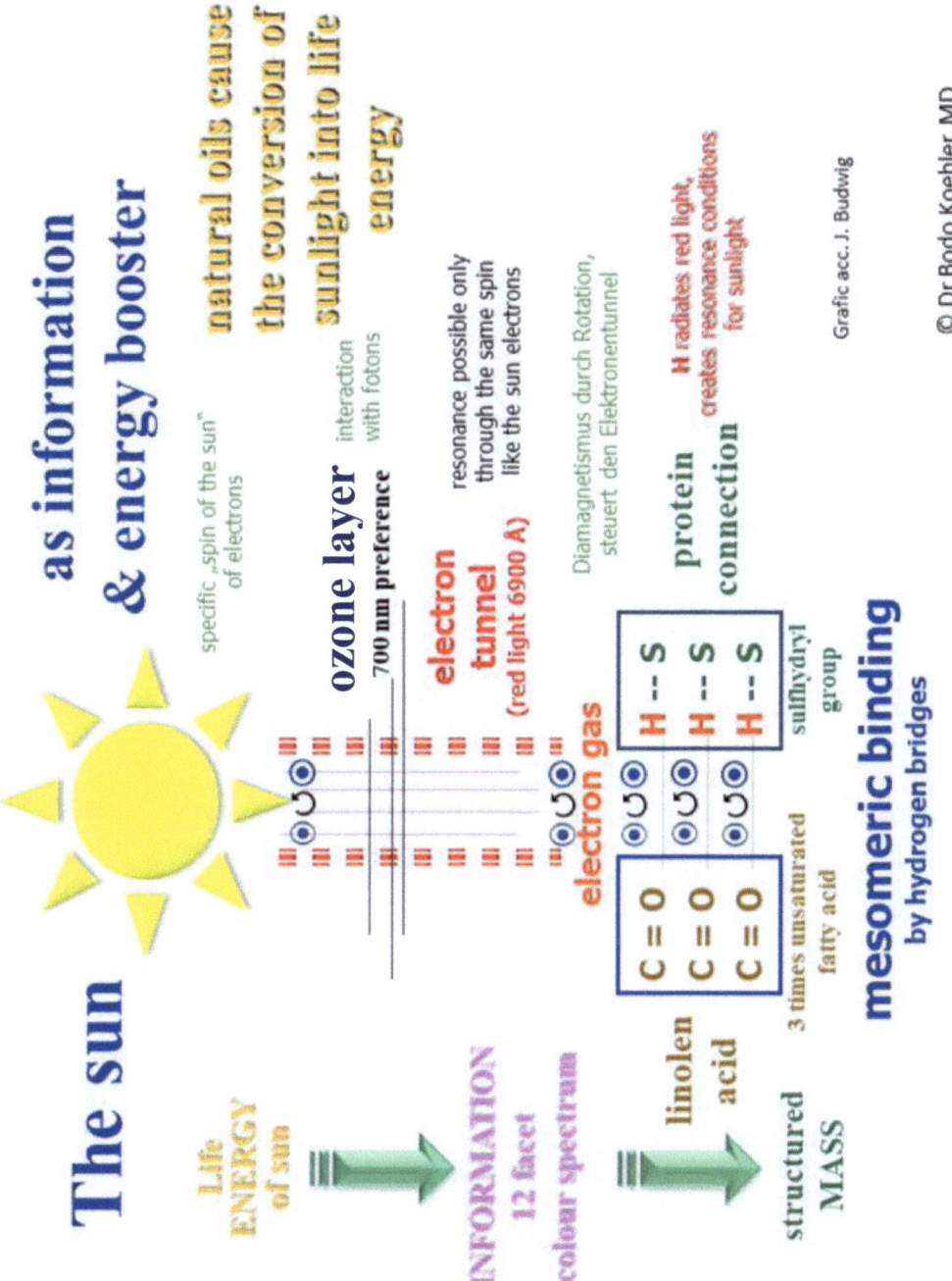

Fig. 3: The source of our life information. Conversion of sunlight into coherent life information and energy in the "solar cells" of the oil-protein compounds

So what mechanisms are at work here?

1. equal spin of the electrons on the sun and in the organism
2. formation of an electron tunnel through diamagnetism
3. red "decoy radiation" of the hydrogen atoms to get into resonance

The last point reflects a universal law that we may encounter more often. "What you fear, you attract." "Your thoughts create your reality." Telepathy also works on this principle. We should therefore be more conscious of our thoughts and words, as we attract all that we think (and fear).

The red radiation is the resonance frequency of the DNA and corresponds to the tone g' (385 Hz). This in turn is the frequency of the earth's rotation (1 / 24 hrs).

It is also important to note that it is primarily not the intensity (strong solar radiation) but the wavelength (red spectrum) that determines how many photons are absorbed (K. Ford). The morning and evening sun is therefore much more favourable and harmless for sunbathing.
As with the visual purple of the eye, the beta-carotene of the carrot is an important mediator for the absorption of photons.

The photons are emitted by us again, but in an altered form. Through the interaction with our organism, they have imparted energy, but also life information to us. After leaving the electrons, they spread the information throughout the body. When they leave the body again, they pick up information about the state of our organism and pass it on.

Information transmission
The transmission of the sunlight in the organism happens via the meridians, which are actively built up via tunnel systems in the matrix (H. Heine). These connect acupuncture points with each other, which in turn have contact with the nervous system. Here the information transmission runs longitudinally via scalar waves (K. Meyl). This is the more highly developed information system that is capable of autoregulation via the brain, which means information processing at a higher level.

Positive electricity combines with heavy matter (has an anabolic effect). Negative electricity (electrons) promotes the dissolution of the same (catabol state). More free π-electron clouds are created.

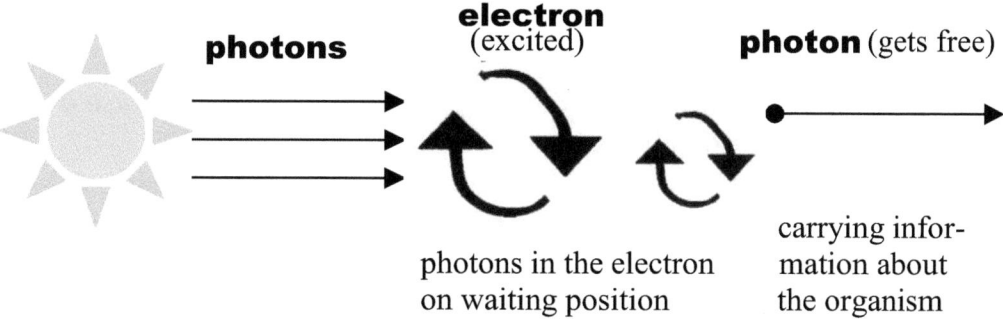

Fig. 4: Electrons as universal light batteries
Human-photon interaction, carrier of life information

According to E. Schroedinger, the "anti-entropy factor" (order-building) in the living organism is based on the ability to attract solar electrons to itself. All life functions are aligned with the sun.

Our structures are adjusted to the sun. Other rays do not resonate with the electrons and cannot be stored as energies.
Winter depression due to lack of light absorption proves this.

H. C. F. Dessauer said: "Man represents on earth the place where light in its transformations in the life process attains the highest concentration of photons."

Photons are the universal energy of the cosmos. They fly with the light, but they are different from it. The human being who is fully charged with them, who lives entirely in their presence, is timeless and lives eternally. Eternity is the now.

The plant is capable of complete photosynthesis. Magnesium and nitrogen are essential for this. Magnesium has 12 protons and 18 steps. The 12th electron has the strongest affinity to photons through its oscillation frequency, which corresponds to f' at base c. Nitrogen has 7 protons and 12 steps.
Magnesium helps to absorb (and re-emit) photons in the green range. Several O_2 molecules also accomplish similar things, e.g. as singlet O_2 or triplet O_2. The ratio of nitrogen to oxygen in the air is about 4 : 1. We find the same ratio in the RNA and DNA base pairs, as well as in the pulse-breath rhythm. O_2 promotes transformation, N_2 stability.

Through its higher development, the human being is dependent on essential substances (e.g. fatty acids), which can go into resonance with sunlight.

Life includes the ability to store sunlight and to be able to release it again at the appropriate time.

Principle of polarity

Since we are not used to thinking in polarities, but rather predominantly in dualities due to the dialectic we have been taught, it is difficult for us to consider the opposite pole at the same time when we speak about a state. But the truth lies hidden in the "both/and", which we can only approach step by step.

If a *clearly expanded* comparison of anabolic and catabolic is listed below, then this is intended to mark the two extremes. Both belong together, are even the same (with the sign reversed). However, it is worth looking at the vertical columns as well. These are correspondences on the different levels of being, *which can all react together*! If there is a disturbance, it can make sense to treat it on another level.

Another aspect is that the two poles are in constant interaction because they are only a different expression of the same thing. They therefore control each other, just as light controls darkness. Darkness cannot exist independently of light.

That which is, that is, our reality, is fundamentally to be understood as polarity. If something comes to the fore, it is only because the other (balancing) pole is weak, is in deficiency.

Symptoms of illness therefore always indicate a (hidden) deficiency that should be sought out and filled. This can show up on different levels and must then also be balanced everywhere. The 3 most important levels are psyche, metabolism and soma.

Everything in our world is polarly, i.e. never without an opposite pole. Sometimes this is not visible at first sight. However, it should always be sought out in order to understand things better. An evaluation of "sunshine" is also only possible with reference to "rain". Only then can correct statements be made. It is the same with illness and health.

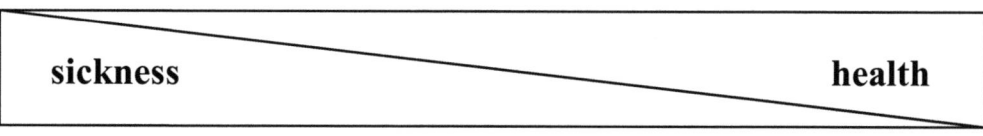

← normal state →

Fig. 5: The polarity of sickness and health

There is no moment in our lives when we are 100% healthy in all areas of our body. There is always "something going on" somewhere, which we call "symptom" or "illness" to distinguish it. This description alone makes it clear that illness is nothing negative at all, but is part of life. Every normal, acute illness must be understood as a healing reaction to ward off any intruders. Only the chronic course brings problems. Then we should go in search of the causes, the blockages, and the *deficiency*.

A very important polarity shows up at the metabolic level:

anabolic	**catabolic**
membranes open	membranes closed
Earth-Water	Fire-Air
mass	energy
corpuscle	wave
rolled-in vortex	rolled-out vortex
photon absorption	photon emission
statics	transformation
visible	virtual
harmonic sounds	noises
bound electrons	free electrons
reducing	oxidising
positive charge	negative charge
coherent light	scattered light
basic valences	acidic valences
magnesium, sodium	calcium, potassium
conservative	progressive
bonding	freedom
Love	individuality
moon	sun
tones	colours
female	male
YIN	YANG

π-Electrons

The secret for health lies in the degree of freedom of the electrons – how many sun photons can be absorbed with the life information they contain. The electrons that are not free, i.e. firmly bound into molecules, convert the messages into structure. In this process, each molecule embodies a specific building block due to its mathematically exactly defined geometry (distances, angles) and ratios (= musical intervals), which can only be used at previously (in the DNA) defined locations (specific localisation).

If localisation shifts occur (e.g. due to trauma), or if there is stress from foreign molecules (pollutants, etc.), then this leads to a weakening of the entire system like a crooked or inverted wall in a house.

The same occurs when stasis occurs during the removal of used substances ("used" means loss of the ability to absorb photons due to contamination with foreign atoms, e.g. mercury) and the burdening substances in this way disturb the "normal operation", i.e. circulation, lymph flow and energy providing.

Health is coupled to the degree of freedom of the π-electrons, which form delocalised electron clouds and can absorb particularly many solar photons, which circle in their tori and carry our life information.

Neutrinos

They have almost become a buzzword, and this is an amazing development that is worth taking a closer look at.

The discovery of this "special particle" is attributed to the Nobel Prize winner Wolfgang Pauli, who only wanted to find a substitute solution for the radioactive beta decay, which had not been completely clarified. He postulated a new particle with certain properties so that physicists could sleep soundly again, but was not convinced of its existence himself.

Years later, however, this "particle" was actually detected and posed new riddles. Actually, it was massless – then it is not a "particle" – but then again it should have some residual mass. It was actually without charge, but behaved as if it had charge, sometimes positive, sometimes negative. Riddle after riddle...

The actual discoverer of neutrinos was Nikola Tesla, a fact that is often kept secret today because Tesla had fallen into disgrace due to his revolutionary ideas. However, he did not use that name. He simply spoke of "radiation".

However, he described the properties of his radiation in the same way as neutrinos are today. In particular, he was already aware of their high penetrating power and that they can move faster (but also slower!) than light.

In atomic physics, the neutrino is the fourth elementary particle (according to the 3 + 1 rule) that belongs to the atom, but on the other hand it does not. It has only a short life span in the nucleus, but a very long one outside of it. Neutrinos can be regarded as the most universal form of energy. They exist in the most diverse forms (also as photons!) and can have very different properties depending on their speed. As a result, they also interact with very different mass structures, depending on where resonant agreement prevails. If the speed of the neutrinos is too high or too low, their energy cannot be used or it can harm us.

The number one elixir of life for us is water, which, due to its various ingredients (minerals or even cells in the blood), each takes on different properties (altered dielectricity) and can therefore interact with different energy states of the neutrinos. There is a special reason why we consist of more than 80% (!) water. It is the inverted primordial sea, which preserves all the life-promoting properties in us that make up our environment, including the resonance conditions for the energy of the neutrinos.

This provides a plausible explanation why certain minerals are necessary for us. Not to be metabolised, but to create the ideal sounding board for the neutrinos.

Blood, saliva, extracellular fluid, lymph, synovial fluid, cerebrospinal fluid, bile and other digestive juices therefore create fundamentally different resonance conditions, resulting in specific functions.

A body fluid by itself could not perform its (active!) biological function at all, since a sufficiently high energy potential is necessary for the enormously high metabolic rate (30,000 to 100,000 chemical reactions per second in each body cell!), which can only be covered by the neutrinos (or their derivatives, the photons).

From this point of view, a new way of looking at toxins and waste products emerges. They change the resonance conditions of the basic structure through their different properties.

Therefore, the importance of the balance of juices is much higher than we usually attach to it. In the case of illness, we should pay increased attention to the composition of the affected fluids.

We can recognise certain characteristics of the liquids:
- **Production and release** (rhythmicity)
- **Fluid composition** (colloids)
- **Intrinsic motion** (leads to induction)
- **Electric field** (charge plus or minus)
- **Magnetic field** (polarity)
- **Spin** (angle and direction of rotation)
- **Potential vortex** (roll-in or roll-out effects)

The therapy goal should be to create optimal resonance conditions for the life-promoting neutrino energy.

Potential vortices

These vortex structures, described and calculated in an outstanding way by Professor Dr Konstantin Meyl, apparently form the basis of all life processes at the electrodynamic level.

Vortices carry a bi-polarity within themselves. Their rolling-in movement is simultaneously opposed by a rolling-out movement. Since they spread out in 3-dimensional space, they simultaneously perform a forward or backward movement perpendicular to it. Their field lines close when rolling in (up to a closed spherical vortex) and open when rolling out (up to their dissolution). Again, the degree of freedom of the *π-electrons* determines the conductivity of the tissue and thus whether the existing potential vortices roll in (anabolic) or roll out (catabolic) and how intensively this happens. Vortices are created by induction, namely when magnetic fields are induced by charge displacement and vice versa. The conditions for this are thus created on the one hand by the existing pi-electron clouds. The intensity with which they form and dynamically oscillate back and forth is an *expression of the life force*, which in turn is metabolically dependent.

With every movement – large and small – they are induced. *Movement* is therefore the second prerequisite for formation. The *strength* of the rolling-in process correlates with the metabolic state. They are subject to the laws of (new) electrodynamics according to K. Meyl.

Potential vortices can be compared figuratively with the wrapping paper of a package. They contain information which they release during the unrolling process. However, they themselves are not the information! Information is a purely mental aspect and therefore physically dimensionless.

Any pressure from outside or even a cold stimulus strengthens the rolling-in process (and thus the closing of the information) up to stable spherical vortices. Here the field lines are closed, the information contained is preserved.

In terms of metabolism (cf. Chapter 5), this would correspond to anabolic derailment.

The release of information occurs in catabolism, which can also be equated with lived individuality.

The conservation of information through the potential vortices means stability, structure and order. The release of the same means renewal, change up to chaos.

All external influences affect the behaviour of the potential vortices – from the psyche to nutrition to certain forms of therapy. Every movement is catabolic, but in the end it has an anabolic effect. This is explained very logically here by the increased curling process caused by this.

Pressure and suction create new vortices, especially in homeostasis, because information can only be absorbed in a meaningful way under constant conditions. The orderly change of pressure and suction creates rhythms – an essential characteristic of homeostasis (cf. H. Heine). This simultaneously determines the frequency of the vortices, or the emitted scalar waves.

The alternation of pressure and suction, i.e. pumping, generates vortices and thus creates an important prerequisite for life.

All fluids are pumped through the organism, but at the same time they provide the counter-impulse through their own movement. This is the only way to explain the functioning of the blood circulation. In purely mathematical terms, the heart would have to accomplish the performance of a cable car every day, which is impossible. Only the vortex theory provides a logical explanation (however, this does not only refer to the fluid vortices – of course, these also play a role – but also to the magnetic and electric potential vortices).

The properties of potential vortices can be described with

- **rolling-in moment** (dynamic)
- **roll-out moment** (always present at the same time, only weaker)
- **frequency** (change between both transitions)
- **direction of propagation** (as scalar wave)
- **stored information** (cannot be measured, only experienced)
- **lifetime** (depending on the metabolic state)
- **amount** (vortex density)

However, they cannot (yet) be measured directly, although this would be of particular importance because it would enable specific statements to be made about the condition of a tissue, a ***universal diagnosis of life***, so to speak.

Through the direct correlation with the dynamics of metabolic regulation, through which the prerequisites for the formation and existence of potential vortices in the organism are created, direct indications of the ***electrodynamics*** in our organism arise. This once again underlines the importance of metabolic measurements as a diagnostic tool.

Disease and health are 2 terms that describe the <u>individual ability</u> to adapt to constantly changing environmental conditions, which requires sufficient energy, vital information and normal regulatory behaviour.

The reasons for a disturbed regulation can be manifold, which carries the danger that the therapist gets lost in details or the patient is sent from specialist to specialist. For this reason it is quite essential to find a ***common basis*** for these functional processes, and that is metabolic regulation (see Chapter 5).

Spiritual-scientific considerations

From a philosophical point of view, there are other interesting aspects that are worth thinking about or that you can simply let sink in.

Photons are not light itself, but they fly with it and are information carriers at the same time. They transmit messages of the mind and possess intelligence (as has been proven in experiments).

According to Max Planck, photons are "very old, immortal intelligences, entities". These are found above all in the ***essence electrons***.

The 4-dimensional reality is linked to the 3-dimensional spirit space by the photon.

Photons are free and individual; otherwise they could not have different wavelengths and vibrate in different frequency ranges, as the 12 colours of light show us. Colours are the language of the spirit. According to Goethe, they are the deeds of light.

Through the absorption of the photons, enlightenment happens in being (matter), whereby transformation becomes possible.

With their entry into matter, either by forming electrons themselves or by energetically exciting already existing ones, they give up their freedom in favour of a strictly ordered structure. They could leave this again, so they are not eternally imprisoned, but they fulfil a very important purpose, which has only become possible by giving up their freedom and individuality - they support life.

Those who are intelligent give up their freedom and give so much good without living their ego, embody pure LOVE.

The stronger the bond, the more love and trust. The more unstable it is, the more freedom and individuality (integration versus separation).

Colours follow the laws of the spirit and are therefore immaterial. Sounds are laws of the spirit that have already become matter and are therefore material. They embody music and mathematics, structure and geometry. They are the blueprint of matter. Through the spirit clothed in phonons (sound quanta), the patterns of life are called up in matter. Every sound, every noise, every tone has structure - from chaotic to highly ordered. There should be no judgement, because everything happens at the right time in the right place, according to a spiritual plan that we cannot see. Through the spirit of time, the realisation of dissolution (transformation) or restructuring (being) takes place.

Tones are "on the spot". The instrument is the atoms on which the phonons play.

In summary, then, the material foundations of life are created by the ***highly unsaturated fats***, in conjunction with proteins and oxygen. The spatial form and orientation necessary for this is made possible by ***standing waves***, which are subject to mathematical-musical laws.
The structure component is formed by the electrons, which are brought into higher states of excitation by photons. These transport spiritual life-

information, because without the creative spirit life would not have come into being and cannot be sustained. This requires an unlimited pool of information.

In order to guarantee the high speed of cell metabolism, a constant supply of energy via **resonant neutrinos** is necessary. The prerequisites for this are created by the **specific composition** of the fluids in the various parts of the body.

The **dynamics** of all processes and in general every movement of our electrically charged organism leads via induction to the formation of potential vortices, which roll in and out depending on the metabolic situation. They can thereby store or release information about the cellular environment.

The normal function of the organism depends on the degree of connection to its environment (cosmos) and the associated level of information (number and character of potential vortices).

On a **spiritual** level, it is the connection to the spirit of God that flows through us as PRANA. For this, the chakras must work harmoniously.

On an **energetic** level, it is electrons that interact with photons and carry life energy (bioplasm – the Qi of the Chinese).

On a **material** level, it is the tones and sounds of the environment (in a negative sense also the noises) as well as all sensory impressions. Internally, it is the normal composition and the free flow of fluids in the vessels as well as in the tissues.

The human organism is a highly dynamic information-processing electrical system whose electrons are in constant interaction with the photons of sunlight, storing and re-emitting them. Man is controlled by soul processes and inspired by the divine spirit.

Even those who have nothing to do with "God" cannot avoid following the quantum physical ideas of a higher intelligence, because without such intelligence, complex life processes are inconceivable.

So if so much effort was made by our creator to put us on two legs, then the whole thing must also have a meaning. Every person will try to find this in his or her own way and come to different conclusions.

However, there is much to suggest that we are on earth in order

- **to gain knowledge through experience**
- **to remember and spread holistic knowledge**
- **to help other people in their development**

Every human being comes into the world with a certain imprint

- **recognisable by the homeopathic miasms**
- **by his individual abilities**
- **his or her unmistakable behaviour**

The sum of all this results in

- **the disposition to disease**
- **the deeper cause of a disease**
- **the part missing for healing, the rejected "shadow".**

He who feels the thirst for knowledge in himself and wants to penetrate deeper into the secrets of life should first familiarise himself with the laws of the universe, because these apply equally outside and inside. In this way he will be spared errors that can have devastating effects in medicine, as we unfortunately have to experience again and again.

3. The Laws of the Universe

After the preceding considerations, summary conclusions can now be drawn about the origin of our reality and thus also of diseases.

materialistic **Natural Science**	spirit-oriented **Holistic Science**
↓	↓
Big Bang	Creation of God
finite universe	infinity
evolution (Darwin)	purpose
closed systems	interactions
self-organisation of matter	intelligent structures

The question therefore arises as to which of the two is able to make scientific statements that best do justice to life processes. The statements of the currently prevailing natural science are sufficiently well known, which is why the focus here is primarily on the spirit-oriented holistic science.

There a top-down direction is followed: From the simple to the complicated, from the idea (of spirit) to the (material) product.

All natural processes, no matter how complicated, are based on very simple principles. These apply everywhere and at all times in the entire universe (macrocosm = microcosm).

Everything was created by spirit. Everything created is spirit.

The meaning: Spirit can only recognise itself in polar reality and attain knowledge through experience.

All bodily structures are subordinate to this goal of cognition!

What is the principle of life?

LIFE is formed through separation – transformation – integration.

For some it may sound too simple that separation and integration should be the basic mechanisms of life. But in every moment of our life we have to make decisions. What is helpful and can be integrated? What could be harmful and should be separated? And this happens on all levels of our BEING. It is therefore worthwhile to take a closer look at this area.

After all, the problems in life begin when it is not recognised that what is rejected comes from the same source as what is preferred, namely from our Creator.

Therefore, our task is not only to take in the positive, but to transform the seemingly negative, to give it a meaning, so that it can then also be integrated.

Constantly rejected areas ("shadows") can materialise into disease foci to demand attention at this level. They bind bioplasm and thus weaken the life energy CHI.

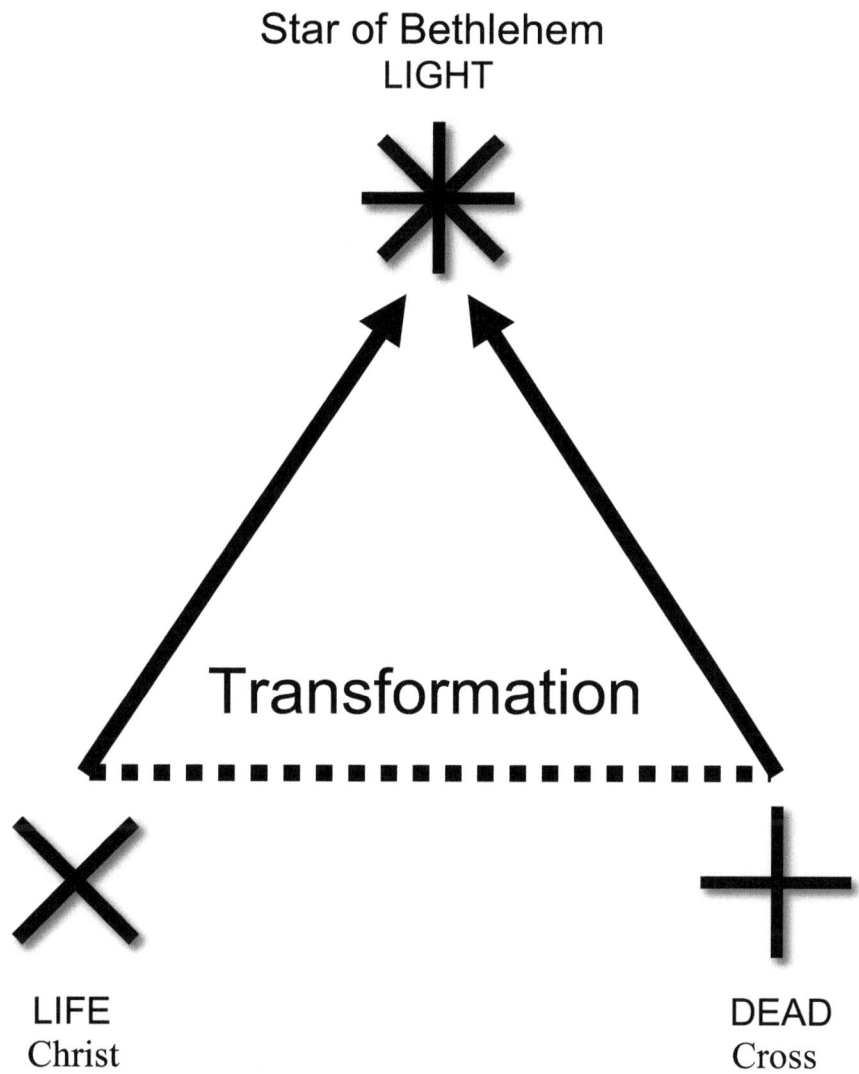

Fig. 6: Separation and integration as a life issue

As will be explicitly explained later in chapter 4, we can understand separation and integration as 2 life axes that are perpendicular to each other. If we want to change something fundamental in our life, then the vernacular speaks of a 180° turnaround. But that would mean that we would have to go back the same way that led us in the wrong direction, which means loss of time. Those who really want to start something fundamentally new should make a 90° turn. This allows us to *immediately* enter new territory and change certain things from the ground up. In concrete terms, this means immediately saying goodbye to everything we have done so far.

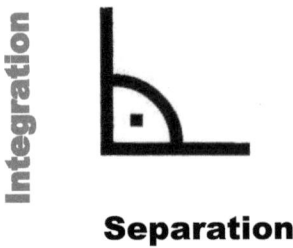

Separation

Fig. 7: Separation and integration as the basic mechanism of life

This immediately shows how difficult it is to actually make a total change in one's life. But already the reorientation, the 90° alignment immediately creates new ideas, new interests and a new attitude to life, whereby the past, to which we are all so attached, quickly fades away. A real sense of optimism can set in, which makes it easier for us to go the new way. Primarily, therefore, our thinking must be oriented differently.

The duality of separation and integration constantly demands decisions for or against life, on all levels of BEING. Lack of decisiveness leads to stagnation in the life process.

The fourfoldness of matter

As already indicated on page 20, there is a strict mathematical blueprint behind our material reality. Nobel Prize winner Wolfgang Pauli (Austrian physicist, 1900-1958) already found the law of the simultaneous 3- and 4-foldness of nature.

According to P. Plichta, the universe is based on number laws. The **3 + 1 rule** found by Pauli will therefore be discussed in more detail.

$$3^4 = 3 \times 3 \times 3 = 81$$

base number 3 = properties   exponent number 4 = control command

There are 81 stable elements (basic building blocks of all matter). This marks the basis of all matter. In its inversion, however, the following formula also has relevance for us:

$$4^3 = 4 \times 4 \times 4 = 64$$

In DNA, 3 bases are combined from 4 possibilities. This results in 64 base triplets. Thus 19 + 1 amino acids are coded (one of the 20, namely glycine, has no asymmetrical centre).

There are also 19 + 1 pure isotopes that have only 1 neutron (one has an odd atomic number). **19 + 81 = 100**

This results in the following interesting relationship:

$4^3 \rightarrow$ **Life processes** (3-fold potentised reality)

$3^4 \rightarrow$ **stability, structure** (4-fold potentised Spirit)

The 3 (trinity of Spirit) controls matter, which always presents itself in a quadruplicity

Max Luescher says to the fourfold "the objective" and to the threefold "the human evaluating". Man is subject and object in one. He therefore obeys the trinity (soul-mind) **and** the quadrunity (structure).

This model shows not only how the two intertwine (matter is spiritualised), but also (on the right-hand side) the dynamics of interactions. Everything is in motion, everything vibrates, but in a 4-fold way. Every impulse leads to a counter-impulse and additionally to movement (rotation) and counter-movement perpendicular to the direction of propagation. This is induction.

As already indicated on page 27, there is a strict mathematical construction plan behind our material reality. Nobel Prize winner Wolfgang Pauli (Austrian physicist, 1900-1958) already found the law of the simultaneous 3- and 4-foldness of nature.

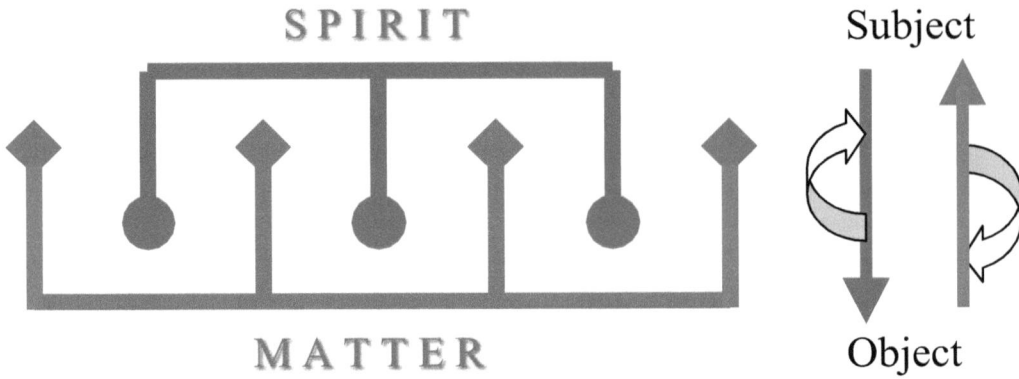

Fig. 8: Spirit-matter interaction and the 4 directions of movement

The numbers can be combined with each other in any way, always resulting in known associations from our material reality.

3	x	4	=	12
Trinity		4 elementary particles		12 human types
		4 DNA bases		12 meridians
		4 miasms		12 colours (Goethe)
		4 seasons		12 tones (+ halves)

3	+	4	=	7
				7 rainbow colours
				7 days of the week
				7-year rhythm
				7 = the human being

The process of materialization

When matter is created, it happens according to an idea of the spirit. Just as every thought can become reality (if the field is strong enough), behind every material structure there is a mental pattern that is reflected in a field. To follow R. Sheldrake, I call it a morphogenetic field, although many authors have used other terms for it. This is also intended to clearly emphasise the transition from the purely spiritual component to the physically verifiable field.

The transition shows itself exactly at the threshold from unity to polarity. Two fields immediately arise that oscillate perpendicular to each other, the magnetic and the electric. Each conditions the other, neither can exist without the other.

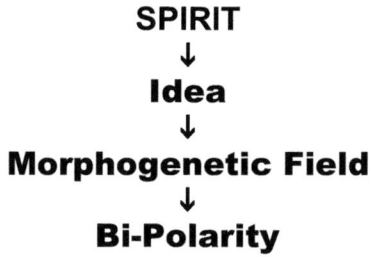

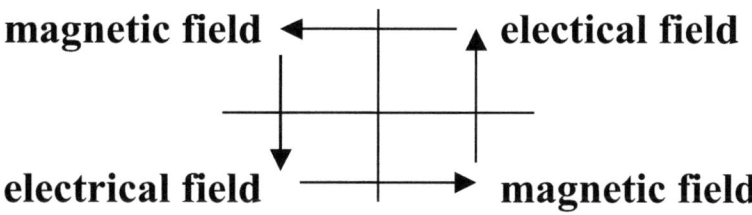

Fig. 9: From Idea to Bi-Polarity

Both planes form a right angle. The one field induces the other. They are merely 2 different manifestations of the spirit, which show themselves through the respective displacement by 90° in a quadruplicity.

The motor for the constant transformation of the fields is attraction and repulsion, sympathy and antipathy. It is therefore a psychological process!

The basis for induction is movement. The law $E = v \times B$ applies (according to M. Faraday) for the electric field and $H = -v \times D$ for the magnetic field.

What do these fields mean, how can we imagine it?

K. Meyl says: "Fields are experiences". He gives the example of a rocket flying through an electric field. It is quite astonishing that the people on board would not feel the electric field, but a magnetic one!

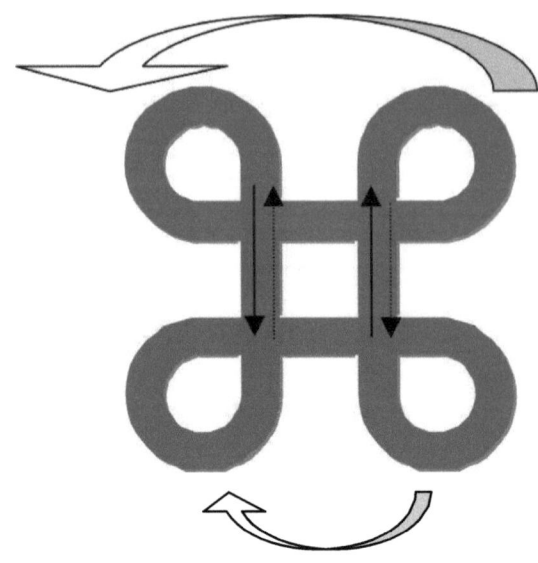

Fig.10: Rotation to the right creates rotation to the left. Each time the 90° angle is passed through, a new quality is created, at 360° there are 4 aspects. At the same time a counter-movement is induced.

You have to think about this calmly for a moment:

Everything we perceive is produced by its opposite. The visible is the product of the invisible.

The fourfoldness is dynamically lived through. Through constant transformation, everything repeats itself and time remains constant (eternity). The return to the starting point should be with new insights, with a higher consciousness. This creates an upward movement (lemniscate). The 4 seasons are examples of this process, but so is the weekly rhythm and the 7-year cycle.

Induction as the motor of transformation

Induction of the counter-movement results in left and right rotation in a ratio of 34 : 21 (Fibonacci sequence). The result is the golden ratio (1.618), the most stable state form of matter.

Up to this point, we can make the following basic observations:

- **A spiritual idea realises itself through fields**
- **Every material phenomenon has 4 forms of state**
- **The visible is based on induction**
- **Life is asymmetry**

The energetic supply of the organism and the supply of information are determined by the **permeability** μ and the **dielectricity** ε. They form a polarity and oscillate back and forth between both extremes.

We distinguish 3 stages:

$\mu\uparrow + \varepsilon\downarrow$ = **superconductivity (catabolic).**
μ - + ε - = **neutral middle**
$\mu\downarrow + \varepsilon\uparrow$ = **vacuum (anabolic)**

As well as 2 additional pathological stages:

$\mu\downarrow + \varepsilon\downarrow$ = **anabolic derailment**
$\mu\uparrow + \varepsilon\uparrow$ = **catabolic derailment**

There are 4 types of movement (3 + 1 - law):

- **longitudinal**
- **transversal**
- **rotation (centrifugal)**
- **vortex with momentum (centripetal)**

The different types of movement also induce different wave patterns, directly depending on permeability and dielectricity. This has far-reaching consequences, which are explained in more detail in chapter 4.

4. The new classification system in medicine

More than 80% chronic diseases, constant increase in medical costs, emergence of new non-treatable diseases, the inflation of therapy offers and other alarm signs should be reason enough to thoroughly rethink today's medical system.

Are there contradictions and if so – what do they look like?

The Human being – a complex, highly dynamic information-processing system

Contradiction no.1:
→ Static investigations (laboratory analyses, imaging methods) do not do justice to this and do not allow any statement to be made about *functional processes*, as they are one-dimensional, without reference to time.

Life is only possible in an open system

Contradiction no.2:
→ Science has not yet succeeded in explaining the phenomenon of "life". The reason lies in the reductionist approach to thinking, instead of an expanded complex view that includes all internal and external interactions. Errors are pre-programmed because the mechanical laws of closed systems are (illicitly) transferred to living organisms.

All organisms have the capacity for self-regulation

Contradiction no.3:
→ This requires intelligent processes to control material structures. Today's natural science proceeds from the materialistic thought of evolution and self-organisation of matter, as a result of which consciousness arises. However, a *spiritual blueprint* is the prerequisite for the emergence of meaningful living structures assigned to specific functions. Spirit creates matter and not the other way round!

Each patient represents a distinctive individual

Contradiction no.4:
→ Therefore he has his own personal medical history. The allocation to *disease groups* does not do justice to this fact in any way. An inadmissible levelling occurs. This is then reflected in a standardised therapy that is laid down in guidelines. This does not require qualified training.

Spirit, soul and body form an inseparable unity with the entire universe

Contradiction no.5:
→ Every analytical division serves to gain knowledge, but is always an artificial division. The more intensive and detailed a diagnosis is, the more it leads away from the actual cause of an illness! This is always to be sought in *disturbed interactions of polar systems* (e.g. anabolic - catabolic).

The list could be continued indefinitely. But this brief overview alone shows that medicine has developed in a completely wrong direction. However, this was not always the case! TCM or Ayurveda, for example, are based on completely different premises. They focus on the life energy as the vulnerable part of our being, in order to be able to intervene here in a corrective way. They are therefore based on completely different systems of order that correspond to Eastern thinking.

Most of the western systems of order used are <u>static</u> and categorise patients according to symptoms. This does not take into account the great dynamics of functional processes in the organism, nor the individuality.

The best way to imagine the difference is that in the Eastern system a complete film is shot of a highly dramatic event (e.g. a thriller), whereas in our Western system a snapshot is taken at any point, from which the entire plot is then inferred.

Classification systems are not only suitable for assigning meaning to seemingly unrelated facts. They also have the task of applying generally valid rules to individual parameters. This means that if one succeeds in classifying something in such a system, then a relationship to the other components can automatically be established and essential correspondences can be found.

Up to now, the order in medicine has been according to diseases. There are superordinate terms, e.g. liver cirrhosis, and all symptoms that fit in with this are subordinated to it. This creates a connection between spider nevi and red palms, as well as to lacquer tongue and oesophageal varices. This sounds good at first. But if the patient suffers from asthma at the same time, then these associated symptoms seem to have nothing more to do with the first and are then assigned to this second disease. Logically, this permanently destroys the unity of the organism.

There is now a completely different way of ordering symptoms. This would consist in leaving the concept of disease as such and starting from the "not healed human being", i.e. the ***deficiency***. This would mean that there is only one problem – instead of many illnesses – namely the individually experienced deficit in the realm of the soul through ***unfulfilled, rejected needs***, resulting from rejection of various aspects of being ("shadow").

This leads us to the question of meaning, which – as we now know from many scientific studies – is essential for us and at the same time determines the course of healing processes. Those who feel useless, who have no task that gives them fulfilment and social recognition, will have little chance of coming out of life crises.

When reorganisation takes place against this background, we arrive at completely different results and, of course, equally new therapeutic approaches. Suddenly, asthma and liver cirrhosis symptoms belong together (anabolic metabolism) as well as the psychic correspondences, the individual choice of colours, peculiarities in the mineral balance, and so on.

In my view, it is therefore an indispensable demand on medicine to revise its overall understanding of life processes. This can best be done by applying systems of order that are geared to this and at the same time have a stable scientific basis and have been tested in practice.

So what are the minimum requirements that these should fulfil?

Classification systems should

1) **obey the mathematical laws of order of the universe**
   (the fourfoldness) **and be 4-dimensional**
2) **take into account the inseparable unity of spirit, soul and body**
3) **show functional relationships**
4) **clarify the interactions among each other**
5) **make hidden causes recognisable**
6) **establish a relationship to other proven systems**
7) **enable a global linkage of all systems of the organism**
8) **bring about a simplification of practical application**
9) **enable a right-brained global overview**

Nine unfulfillable demands? That's how it seems at first glance. The impression is deceptive. Such a system has already existed for 70 years, but is only now slowly coming to full bloom due to the multitude of new findings from the most diverse fields of holistic science.

However, in order to learn to appreciate the value of such a model, it is necessary to derive it and to relate it to other (ancient) systems, with which it is already possible to work quite well, at least in 2 dimensions.

The 4 elements

The Greek Empedocles – who lived 2500 years ago – is credited with founding the 4 elements doctrine. However, it is more likely that people in earlier advanced civilisations already knew this system, since it is the ***original principle of whole creation***.

This is only now slowly coming to consciousness since P. Plichta produced the mathematical derivation of the basic structure of the universe, which is based on the numbers 3 and 4. In the past, people were much more connected to nature than they are today. They observed the stars, the moon, the sun and the course of the seasons – simply everything around them, because they tried to live in harmony with nature. So certainly the fourness as a law inherent in matter was known much earlier.

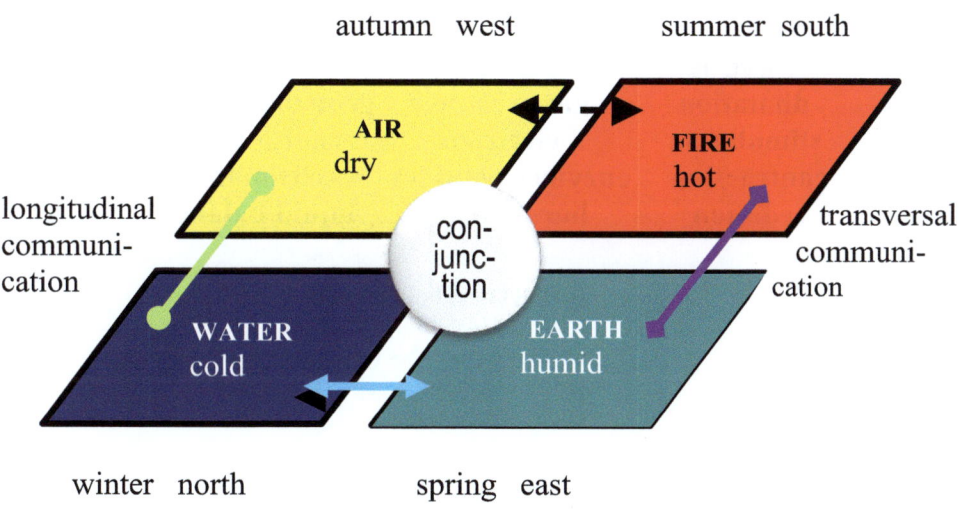

Fig.11: The system of the 4 elements. Air is the master of fire (fires up). Fire warms the air. Water is the master of the earth (keeps it moist), but is guided by it (riverbed, bank).

The 4 elements are in constant interaction, whereby a temporal circulation to the left results (as with the seasons). At the same time, however, a counter-movement is induced to the right. This is quite understandable. In winter there are often very warm "summer" days and, conversely, very cold days in summer, including hailstorms.

All BEING is produced by its opposite and produces its opposite again.

According to C. G. Jung, the sphere in the middle represents the conjunctio, or as we will see later, the life - s - light, the point of connection of all 4 elements. This is where the interactions between them are experienced. This is where the observer, or the subject, the patient or we, is/are located. This closes the circle to the Chinese teaching of the 5 transformation phases, which can easily be misunderstood if the process is only considered on one level.

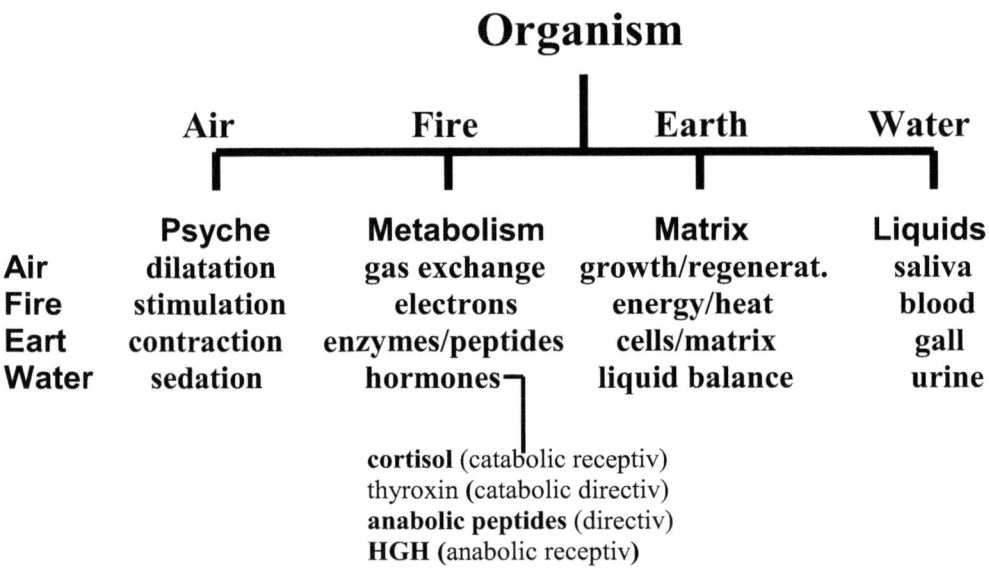

Organism

	Air	Fire	Earth	Water
	Psyche	**Metabolism**	**Matrix**	**Liquids**
Air	dilatation	gas exchange	growth/regenerat.	saliva
Fire	stimulation	electrons	energy/heat	blood
Eart	contraction	enzymes/peptides	cells/matrix	gall
Water	sedation	hormones	liquid balance	urine

cortisol (catabolic receptiv)
thyroxin (catabolic directiv)
anabolic peptides (directiv)
HGH (anabolic receptiv)

Fig. 12: The Quadrity(ies) of Life

It is incredibly exciting once you delve into this system and try to experience the world around you in its fourfoldness. Only then are "objective" observations possible. All phenomena in reality occur 4-fold. If we recognise only 2 or 3 aspects, we should look for the missing ones, otherwise we will not get a real picture of reality. This is the basis of most misunderstandings.

Open System Human

			PRANA	Posture-
Air	$\rightarrow$	**breath (O_2, N_2) Qi**		**inform.**
			rhythm	**movement**
			photons	Life-
Fire	$\rightarrow$	**sun light**	**Qi**	**inform.**
			neutrinos	**energy**
			resonance	Uptake of
Earth	$\rightarrow$	**structures**	**Qi**	**inform.**
			sound	**transform.**
			vitality	Toroid-
Water	$\rightarrow$	**information**	**Qi**	**structures**
			vortex	storage

$\downarrow$ $\qquad$ $\downarrow$ $\qquad$ $\downarrow$ $\qquad$ $\downarrow$

Rapid adaptability to changing environmental conditions

Interactions with all levels of BEING

Development of consciousness with gain of knowledge through experience

Life-enhancing, responsible action through new insights

When we talk about coming into balance, this concretely means having an undisturbed relationship with all 4 elements – none will be preferred, none rejected. For example, if you say that you can't stand cold, you reject the water element, which corresponds to the relaxing blue, and then look for the following as a substitute (as compensation) activity (red) or even distraction (yellow) instead of seeking the cause of the lack of energy (catabolic blockage). This can very quickly lead to serious kidney problems.

This closes the circle: life is only possible in the long run if it itself contributes to supporting life processes.

The Luescher Cube

Let us now turn to the 4-dimensional system of **regulatory psychology,** the **Luescher cube**. This was first introduced by Prof Dr Max Luescher in 1953 and initially referred to the colour assignments to mental disorders. In recent years, he himself attempted an interdisciplinary analysis, which led to further assignments. Thus he added the miasms of homeopathy, as well as the single remedies themselves.

35 years ago, the author has succeeded in impressively underpinning the general validity of the model by adding a significant extension through the classification of the groundbreaking findings on metabolic regulation according to Prof Dr Dr Juergen. Schole (three-component theory). In addition, the most important minerals, which are essential for the function of the matrix, were included, as well as the main groups of nutrition.

A completely new impulse now came from electrodynamics. Already J. Schole had described metabolic regulation as an electron-donor-acceptor reaction. Life – and thus health and performance – take place in a rhythmic alternation of resting potential (anabolic) and dynamic electron flow at the wall-bound flavin radicals (catabolic). Therefore, the research results of Prof Dr Konstantin Meyl now fit seamlessly into the system, which simultaneously demonstrated the coherence of both disciplines – metabolism and electrodynamics.

But this is by no means the end of the story. It is only the beginning of a completely new understanding of medicine, which on the one hand means a significant simplification of medicine (from the whole to the detail, instead of the other way round) and on the other hand enables ***direct access*** to the hidden cause of disease, but without extensive diagnostics!

At the same time, this ordering system of Life-supporting Medicine LSM represents a model with which diagnostic or therapeutic systems can be checked for their correctness, and furthermore, even scientific predictions are possible!

Now it is possible to start establishing connections to other holistic systems (they have already been mentioned in part earlier), which will sooner or later lead to a unification of the whole of medicine. After all, there is only one medicine that can really be optimally applied in individual cases – a small selection from many therapeutic possibilities that is best tailored to the individual human being who stands before us as a patient. The rapid realisation of this goal has now become possible through the practical application of the 4-dimensional ordering system to *Life-supporting Medicine*.

With the Luescher cube, there is quite obviously a model that depicts the universal principles of life and on which the interactions of the individual components can be shown.

The cube model is of great practical use, because it can be implemented immediately on the patient. Above all, the true, underlying cause of a health disorder can be grasped at a glance.

But it is only by deriving this system that the four-dimensionality becomes comprehensible.

Max Luescher starts from two basic behaviour patterns (constellation) of the psyche in the **1st dimension**. They are **directive** and **receptive**. They are polar opposites and can also be experienced in their exaggeration (++) as **suggestible** versus **authoritarian**.

Perpendicular to this we have the **2ⁿᵈ dimension**, which is composed of **variable** and **constant**. In its exaggeration (++) we experience it as **unsteady** versus **fixed**.

Both axes can be shifted against each other at will, so that, as in real life, one acts and reacts more with constant vigour, the other more passively and wait-and-see. From each of the 2 components result in the 4 basic structures of the psyche, which in turn form polarities: **Dilation** and **contraction**, as well as **stimulation** and **sedation**. These are represented by the **4 Luescher colours**.

The horizontal "experience level" is thus represented as follows:

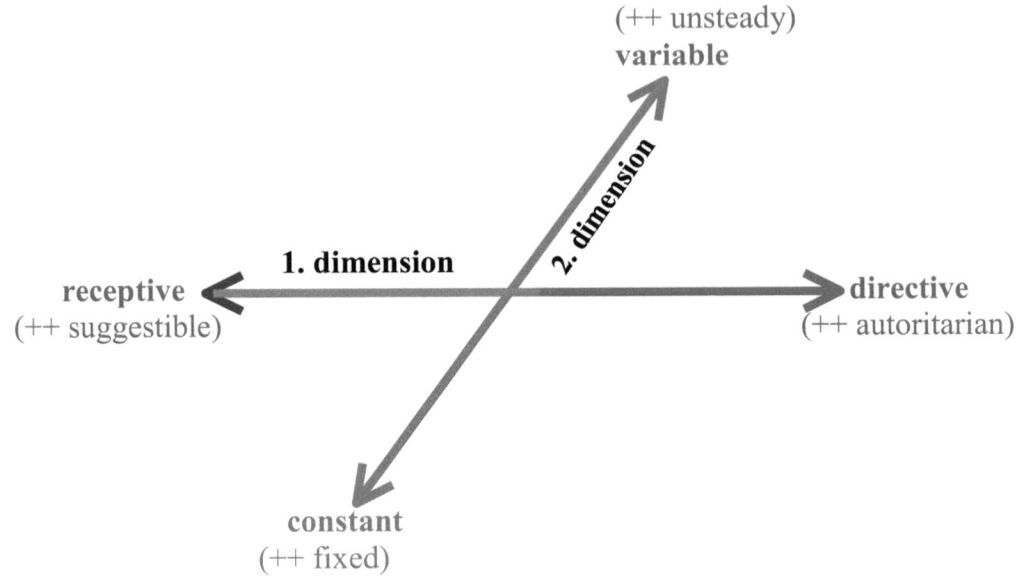

Fig.13: Object – Subject – Relation of the Human

Constant-receptive becomes calming **dark blue**, **constant-directive** becomes strengthening dark **green-blue**, **variably-directive** becomes active **red-orange** and **variably-recep**tive becomes liberating **yellow**.

At the same time, these results in the **3rd dimension**, which is represented by the diagonals. Yellow and green stand for **separation** (differentiation), blue and red for **integration**. This already brings us to our principle of life. You have to imagine it in such a way that through the constantly necessary decisions that we have to make between the two, a passing through all 4 aspects takes place in order to illuminate reality from all sides. So we rotate around the centre, with the centre indicating the balance of our behaviour, the *middle*.

Through the experiences we have in the process, our knowledge increases and we begin to value and evaluate. Our life is decisively determined by this. We thus determine ourselves, preferring certain areas and rejecting others. Thus we leave our centre downwards or upwards, which is made clear by the vertical axis, the **4th dimension**. This creates a tri-polarity.

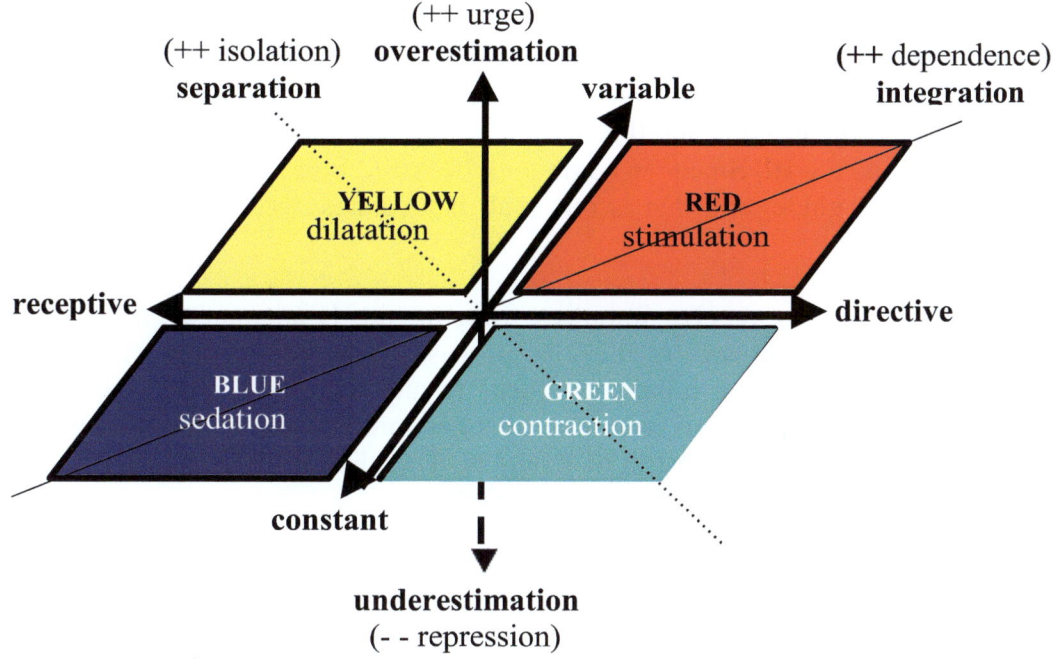

Fig. 14: Integration-Separation and Estimation (4. Dimension)

Excessive (- -) **underestimation** leads to **repression**, to the suppression of important aspects of life, which results in *lack*. Out of this resulting dissatisfaction, an attempt is made to compensate for this deficit. An **overestimation** of other aspects takes place, which can increase to an **urge** (++), e.g. addiction.

As we will see later, the development of the disease can be read from this vertical axis. The superficial symptom will show up "above" in the area of overvaluation in *compensation.* The cause, however, is to be sought "below" in the suppression.

This rejected aspect of life is called the "shadow". It is the suppressed needs. On the *metabolic level* this corresponds to the blockage of anabolic or catabolic, on the *physical level* to the invisible underlying cause which (delocalised!) produces the symptom and corresponds to the *constitutional weak point (CWP)*. This conforms to the *homoeopathic miasm*.

This previous section describes the decisive connections of every disease development! Therefore, the functional levels mentioned will be described in more detail.

Under the viewpoint (of quantum mechanics) that life could and can only be created by a higher intelligence, there must also be a meaning behind it, a life task, a goal. Since we come into the world blind, so to speak, we need a constant guide, and that is our soul. It mediates between spirit and matter (body).

We constantly receive impulses from it, mostly in images, reinforced by sensations in the area of the solar plexus, which show us the way. Unfortunately, the rational mind often steps in and interposes misgivings. This is supposed to protect us from imprudent actions, but often leads to a blockade in people with a head full of thoughts. This disturbs personal development, because new stimuli are always needed.

The resulting dissatisfaction with the course of life so far is attempted to be compensated for by substitute satisfactions, alcohol or drugs. Those who pass by their lives in this way do not act according to their constitution and can easily overexert themselves. The genetically inherent weak points (CWP) in every human being come under stress. In order to avoid a derailment, these areas are "walled in" with *bioplasm*, which leads to an increased consumption of essence electrons. These photons, charged with life experience and circling in the electron tori, are missing in other places and weaken the overall system "human being".

The first step towards healing would therefore be to release blockages by releasing fears, making peace and then starting a new life with joy, with "desire for something new", which corresponds to the Luescher yellow. This is not so easy. But with the right background knowledge, the necessary expansion of consciousness can take place better.

In order to be able to carry out this assignment according to the colours, a complete Lüscher test is necessary. Compensation (++) and cause (- - = rejected part) can be read from the multiple selection of the same colours (columns). The measured current metabolic situation then corresponds to the compensation, expressed by ++.

69

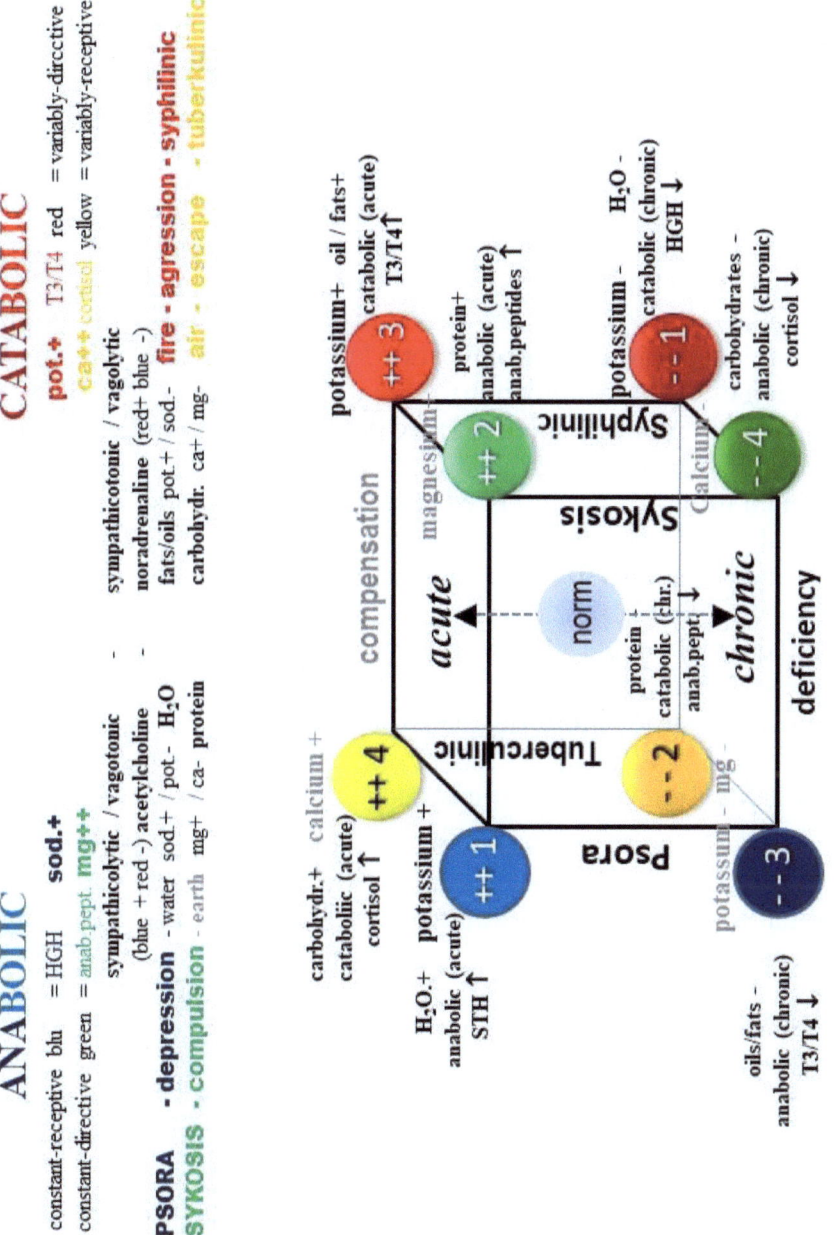

Fig. 15: Nutrition, Minerals, Miasms & Metabolic Regulation

©Dr Bodo Koehler, MD

The classification in the Luescher cube makes it possible to recognise, among other things:

1) Where is the actual cause of the disease (= deficiency)?

For this purpose we orientate ourselves on the lower 4 corners (- -) (Fig. 15):

- Which **genetic** disposition (genotype) is present?
  (expressed by the homeopathic miasm = edge of the cube)
- What is the **basic psychoenergetic structure** present? (variable-constant in interaction with receptive-directive).
- What is rejected on **psycho-level**? (calm - firmness - activity - opening)
- What is the **initial metabolic state**? (anabolic or catabolic, gives indication of counter-regulation)
- Which **hormones** (regulators) are deficient? (with indication of insufficient endocrine glands)
- Which **minerals** are involved? (the minus sign at the bottom expresses the deficiency)
- What are the **nutritional** deficiencies? (carbohydrates - water - fats - protein)
- Is there a **distorted view of reality** (underestimation)? (Assignment to the self-esteems)
- Which **dream symbol** fits the basic problem?

2) How is the deficiency compensated?

For this we orientate ourselves on the upper 4 corners (++) of Fig. 15:

- What is the **current metabolic state**? (Leads to the predominant symptoms)
- Which **regulators** (metabolic hormones) are dominant?
- Which **electrolytes** are in excess?
- Which **foods** are in excess?
- How is compensation on the **psycho level**? (Addictions - arrogance – show-off - illusion)

According to M. Luescher, the development of a *neurotic maladjustment* takes place in easily comprehensible steps, which can be traced on the Luescher cube:

- **misjudgement of reality, disturbed perception**
- **egocentric, unreal, illusionary exaggerated demands (++)**
- **fear that they will not be fulfilled (- -)**

ASSIGNMENTS

blue constant- receptive	green constant- directiv	red variably- directive	yellow variably- receptive
calm	firmness	activity	opening
– – self- dissatisfact.	rejection: self- doubt	self- regret	– – self- compulsion
+ + addictions	compensation: arrogance	show-off	+ + illusion
anabolic **HGH**	**anabolic** **peptides**	**catabolic** **thyroxin**	**catabolic** **cortisol**
Psora	Sycosis	syphilinic	tuberculinic
depression	compulsion	aggression	escape
sodium	magnesium	potassium	calcium
water	protein	fats/oil	carbohydr.
sympathicolisis	vagotonic	sympathicotonic	vagolysis

Table 1: Assignment according to the quadruplicity (Luescher/Koehler)

Through the rejection of true reality, egocentrically exaggerated demands and illusions (++ = heaven) follow, which can lead to an acute illness (= derailment of a chronic initial situation = deficiency).

The best way to demonstrate these complex relationships is with a concrete example from practice.
Imagine a young allergy sufferer (18 years) with the leading symptom hay fever, which manifests itself very violently and persistently. In his behaviour, the patient seems calm, rather adapted and almost sleepy.

He tends to reject "modern things". He lacks initiative to a large extent, as well as determination. He lives in the day. His metabolism is + 50° anabolic. The Luescher test shows (in the columns) ++1 (blue preferred) and - -2 (green rejected).

Then we find the following correlations (cf. Fig.15):

- *Blue preferred* (urge for rest and satisfaction, addictions)
- *Metabolic state acutely anabolic* (increased membrane permeability, therefore swollen mucous membranes with all consequences = ++1)
- *HGH increased* (in relation to cortisol and T3/T4 low)
- *Sodium increased* (can also be relative potassium deficiency)
- *Too much water* (eat less water-rich foods)
- *Green rejected* (evasive, vegetatively unstable)
- *Chronic anabolic basal metabolism* (with acute phase)
- *Low anabolic peptides* (no reserves, recovery needed = - -2)
- *Lack of magnesium* (relative calcium surplus possible)
- *Lack of protein* (should avoid carbohydrates)
- *Receptive receiving* (passive, as opposed to directive doing)
- *Self-doubt* (lack of self-respect)
- *Dream symbol the agile snake* (stands for adaptation)

Tuberculinic indicates *weakness*, **Psora** depression, **Sycosis** *compulsion* and **syphilinic** *aggression*. All this can be read on the Luescher cube. It takes only a few minutes to do this.

There are far-reaching consequences for therapy:

- **Metabolic balancing with SRT, ZMR. MRT, MORA***nova*
- **Colour-tone therapy with green and blue** (alternating)
- *Integration of the shadow* (corresponds to green)

- *Stepping out of passivity into activity*
- *Reduction of one's own overestimation* (reduction of addictions)
- *Creating self-respect* (through a sense of achievement)
- *Avoidance of carbohydrates* (in the acute phase)
- *Supply of wholesome protein* (no sugar!)
- *Building up reserves through rhythms* (interval training)
- *Adherence to regular breaks* (order)
- *High doses of magnesium*
- *Avoiding table salt*

This clearly shows that the *allergens* as such do not play a primary role in the patient, but take a back seat in the holistic thinking. The main reason for pollinosis in this patient is insufficient self-respect due to undervaluation of the self.

The recommendation to the patient would be: *Realise your own ideas with seriousness in order to promote self-esteem through a sense of achievement.*

So we always have to orient ourselves on the lower level (- -), because the deficiency should be filled up. If we start here causally, real healing can be achieved. *Causal* means here (as basically in life-supporting medicine) treatment on all 3 levels of BEING *at the same time*. This means not only an end to the symptoms of the illness, but a leap in development through a gain in knowledge. Then an illness has also fulfilled its *purpose*.

Once the principle has been understood and integrated into the practice, we have an instrument at our disposal that not only enables complex observations on the development of illness. It can also be read off how the individual findings have to be assigned and whether the therapy regime is coherent in itself, i.e. works synergistically.

There are also new complex ways of looking at the *conflict structures*, in connection with the metabolic situation.

These are determined by the columns in the Lüscher test. On the left side, the preferred parts are sought out (which are to be understood as compensation for the rejected ones). On the right are the psychostructures that are not lived. It should be noted that the left area results from the right, i.e. is the consequence of an avoidance strategy (shadow).

Conflict structures

(correspond to the connections of the corners in the cube)

yellow axis:	++ 4 **illusion, escape** dilated, collapse **acute catabolic** **cortisol** ↑	- - 4 **apprehension, anxious** constricted, tightness **chronic anabolic** **cortisol** ↓
red axis:	++ 3 **aggressivity** irritable **acute catabolic** **thyroxin** ↑	- - 3 **resignation** exhausted **chronic anabolic** **thyroxin** ↓
blue axis:	++ 1 **urge for rest** and satisfaction **acute anabolic** **HGH** ↑	- - 1 **discontentedness, restlessness** agitated **chronic catabolic** **HGH** ↓
green axis:	++ 2 **arrogant** tense **acute anabolic** **anab. peptides** ↑	- - 2 **evasive** vegetatively unstable **chronic catabolic** **anab. peptides** ↓

So if, as in the above example, ++1 is chosen, it is only because green, i.e. No. 2, is rejected. The cause therefore lies in the lack of self-respect, the rejection of seriousness and the lack of inner stability. So that is where we have to start. The weaker part should always be supported and not the dominant one fought against.

One can see very clearly that with the conflict structures on the right side there is always a deficiency situation in the area of hormones. This can mean that too few hormones are being secreted (which is especially important with to be taken into account with HGH). But it can also be an indication of exhaustion of the corresponding hormone gland. In the latter case, it must be actively supported, possibly even through temporary hormone substitution; otherwise no normalisation of the metabolism and thus healing is possible.

The behaviour, the ethical control, results from the self-esteem (the self-control according to Max Luescher).

self-esteems			**ethical control**		
blue	-	contentedness	**blue**	-	personal contentedness
green	-	serious	**green**	-	self-respect
red	-	vividness	**red**	-	self-confidence
yellow	-	serenity	**yellow**	-	personal freedom

However, the Luescher test also attaches special importance to indifferent, non-rejected colours. This is the "normality". This aspect is not questioned. That is just the way one is. When change is demanded, it should be kept in mind that this is the reason for the full satisfaction, for the habit that will always stand in the way of a process of rethinking.

Even the most targeted psychotherapy will not be successful if the conditions on the body level are not met. Profound changes need prolonged crises! Without chronic stress there is no acute illness.

However, this is hidden in the background. The superficial symptom tends to distract from it. The Lüscher colours now provide direct access.

In summary, it can be said that with the classification of the basic components of cell metabolism in the 4-dimensional Luescher cube, a new chapter in medicine has begun. Here, mathematical-geometrical laws meet with the basic building blocks of life, which are responsible for structure and functional processes. At the same time, the cube model shows that time itself does not represent the 4th dimension, but is superordinate.

The diagonal in the cube (between ++ and - -) shows the life axis onto which all events are projected, as well as the actions controlled by the self-esteems as a reaction to them, via the hormonal regulators. Since hormones are the messenger substances of the soul, the missing link between psyche and soma, the missing dimension, was found, through which a holistic view of the human being becomes possible.

5. Metabolism regulation and its importance

Even if it sounds unfamiliar to some ears at first: The regulation of the cell metabolism has the highest priority in all of medicine! *All* therapeutic procedures must be measured by their influence on the cell metabolism. Whether it is conventional medicine that is applied, naturopathic treatments or psychotherapy – if it does not succeed in positively influencing an entrenched, derailed metabolic situation, the chosen method is not suitable for the patient.

With the measurement of the cell metabolism regulation, we have an instrument in our hands with which the effectiveness of a therapy method can be proven directly on the patient on a very individual basis.

That is something very special. But it goes even further. We can also use it to carry out excellent follow-up checks and preventive examinations. Regulatory rigidity can be identified through multiple measurements or a provocation test. From the measured metabolic situation, very specific dietary recommendations can be derived and at the same time compliance with dietary regulations can be monitored.

All this gives cell metabolism regulation its central role in medicine. It is not only the link between all disciplines, but also brings together orthodox medicine and complementary medicine, because both must be oriented towards the effects on the patient. *Cell metabolism is the general frame of reference.*
Fig.16 shows very clearly that all areas of medicine and daily life are grouped around cell metabolism regulation, thus forming a cohesion, a reference platform. If you take out this central part, everything else hangs incoherently in space. This is the situation we find ourselves in today, which is further reinforced by the expansion of specialism. What we lack is the unifying, the connecting element, the general system of reference.

Every chronic disease is the expression of a derailment of the cellular metabolism with loss of adaptability, either locally or generally.

The reason for this can lie at all levels. If a permanent mental problem has led to stagnation in the life process, this is just as relevant for a metabolic derailment as an energetic deficit due to the lack of π-electrons (bioplasma) and the associated depletion of sun photons. However, extensive destruction of necessary tissue components can also be responsible, especially of the highly sensitive lipoid membrane structures, combined with a drastic drop in the degree of order in the tissue (entropy), which has an unfavourable effect on the transmission of information. We find this situation in all chronic inflammations up to cancer.

The cell environment system

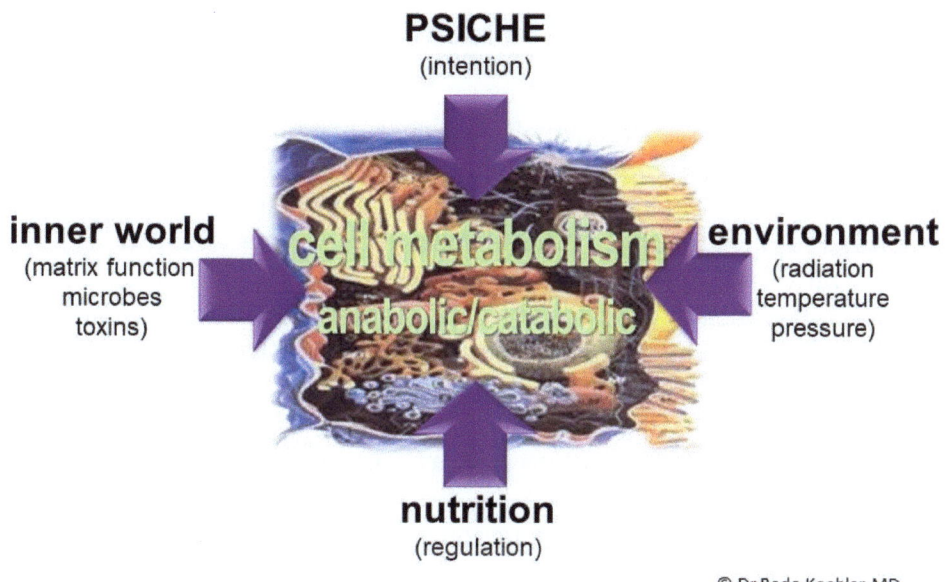

© Dr Bodo Koehler, MD

Fig. 16: The central position of cell metabolism regulation in medicine

Understanding the regulation of cell metabolism therefore offers a great opportunity to finally overcome the fragmentation caused by specialism, the dispute over methods between the different views, as well as the growing unmanageability of medicine. Learning to be a doctor and classifying the various symptoms of a patient could be made much easier. It is therefore worthwhile to study the basics more closely.

Metabolism
What is meant by this?
If we ask the patient about a metabolic disorder, he usually thinks of his digestion. If we talk to a colleague, it is usually about diabetes. Nobody really knows surely what is meant by metabolic regulation.

At this point it should also be pointed out that even in the "official" opinion (of the specialists) on metabolic regulation there are a lot of inconsistencies. One reason is the previous assumption that metabolic processes would be slowed down or accelerated by conversions from anabolic to catabolic enzymes and vice versa – in which co-enzymes play a role (allosteric influence of phosphofructokinase). This was called the *Pasteur Effect*. According to today's knowledge, however, the Pasteur Effect is primarily dependent on the *redox status of the cell* and can also become *negative*. It is therefore defined today as a "change in the rate of synthesis by varying the O_2 partial pressure, while the enzyme concentration remains constant".

High O_2 partial pressure (which, however, is caused by oxygen *suction* (!) due to the *auto-oxidation* of highly unsaturated fatty acids) means a high concentration of electron acceptors for the respiratory chain and thus increased ATP formation. Anabolism and thus growth, anti-body formation etc. requires the inhibition of the "Pasteur Effect". This is achieved by the anabolic peptides in the cells. The connection metabolism – matrix is made by the supply of nutrients. If the molecular sieve is not permeable, there is no anabolic growth.

The glutathione system can be seen as a mirror image of the redox system with seamless interconversion (to be understood as division of labour). Direct connections with the functional state of the immune system can be seen here. But more on this later.

Basic regulation

The anabolic synthesis and the catabolic energy metabolism are interrelated and mutually dependent. Neither can be correctly described without simultaneous consideration of its partner (YIN-YANG principle). Their activity is the same at rest. It is ensured by the so-called basic regulation, which is characterised by oxidation and reduction processes, by the exchange of electrons (electron donor-acceptor reactions), a constant giving and giving back. The redox potential determines the basic regulation and thus ensures the "everyday metabolism" of the cells.

Understanding the regulation of cell metabolism therefore offers a great opportunity to finally overcome the fragmentation caused by specialism, the dispute over methods between the different views, as well as the growing unmanageability of medicine. Learning to be a doctor and classifying the various symptoms of a patient could be made much easier. It is therefore worthwhile to study the basics more closely.

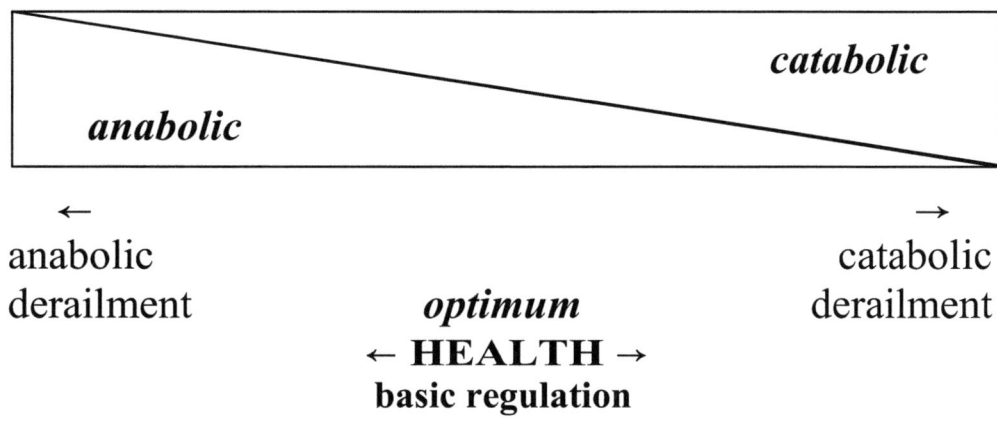

anabolic
derailment

optimum
← **HEALTH** →
basic regulation

catabolic
derailment

Fig. 17: The polar principle of cell metabolism regulation

If one considers that 30,000 to 100,000 chemical reactions take place in each cell per second (!) (this are 10^{18} reactions per second in the entire organism – an unspeakably large number), then the question of intelligent, sufficiently fast control naturally arises. In purely mathematical terms, the reactions must be triggered within 1 nanosecond (10^{-9} seconds). Only ***photons*** coming from the DNS transmitter – receiver system are capable of this. Their laser-like impulses control these processes. Photons bring electrons into higher orbits (excited state), making them more reactive with neighbouring atoms. This means that the basic regulation can take place without, or only with minimal, activation of hormones.

If stimulus loads occur – this can be stress, but also a load from toxins, microbes, viruses, etc. – then the higher-level hormonal regulators must step into action more strongly in order to bring about an appropriate adaptation to the load as quickly as possible. In this process, not both metabolic parts are "ramped up" at the same time, but one after the other. It is the time delay, the "lagging behind", that is the disease value. In a rested state – with appropriate reserves of cortisol and anabolic peptides – the balance at a higher energetic level is already achieved after 1 hour (!). Otherwise it takes 4-5 days and usually runs with the symptoms of an acute illness (which must be understood as a healing reaction!) corresponding to the "alarm reaction" according to Selye.

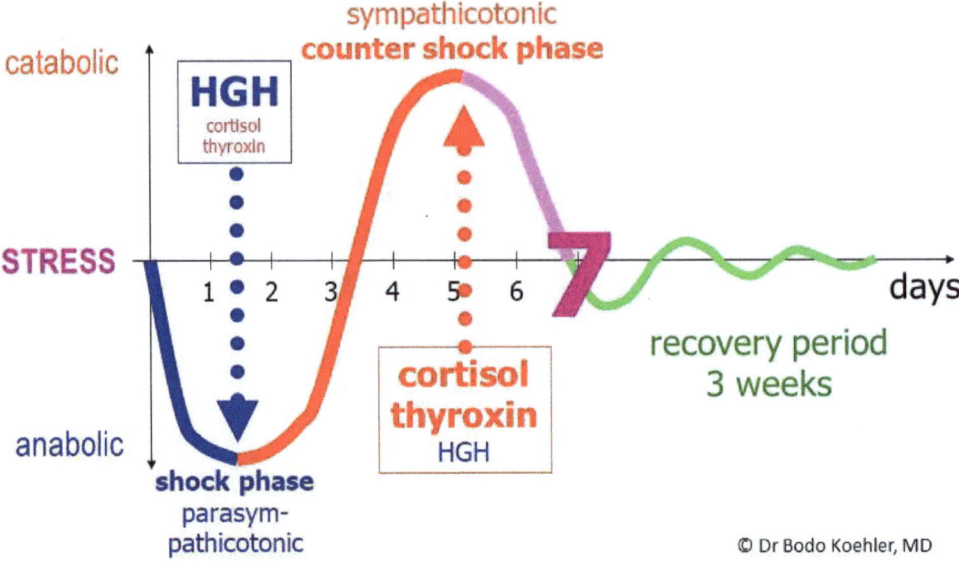

Fig. 18: Alarm reaction phases of the metabolism acc. to H. Selye

First, a "shock phase" is run through, which is parasympathicotonic and thus *anabolic*, and then on the third day it changes to the sympathicotonic "counter-shock phase", which is *catabolic*. After exactly one week, the process (the acute healing reaction) is usually completed. This is followed by a three-week "convalescence phase".

The acute anabolic phase is characterised by the classic inflammatory signs rubor, tumor, calor, and dolor. The functional characteristics are besides a *high production rate of antibodies* an *increased membrane permeability*. There is increased leakage of fluid into the tissue with all the consequences. The patient usually has a high fever, but feels cold (chills), tired and apathetic.

The transition to the catabolic counter-shock phase is associated with a drop in fever on the third day, but severe heat and sweating. The patient is usually restless. After one week, the symptoms have disappeared. What remains is a certain weakness. However, there is a risk of relapse on the 8th day!

This can lead to symptoms again, which should definitely give cause for a follow-up treatment. Otherwise, a gradual progression (e.g. Post Covid) or a massive aggravation can occur. This can be easily controlled with Living Systems Information Therapy (LSIT), but only if the alarm reaction is known and intervention takes place immediately on the 8th day.

Complications of this kind only occur if the shock phase according to Selye cannot be fully acted out, i.e. if the healing high fever is missing or suppressed, which is unfortunately the standard of orthodox medicine.

Ignorance about metabolic regulation can cost lives!

It also becomes pathological when the patient gets stuck in the catabolic phase.

Three component regulation

According to J. Schole, metabolic regulation can only take place if 3 components are in use *simultaneously* as so-called "basic regulators": **Thyroid hormones** and **cortisol** (activate the flavin enzymes in the mitochondria and therefore have a catabolic effect), and **HGH** or the **anabolic cell peptides** (inhibit the flavin enzymes).

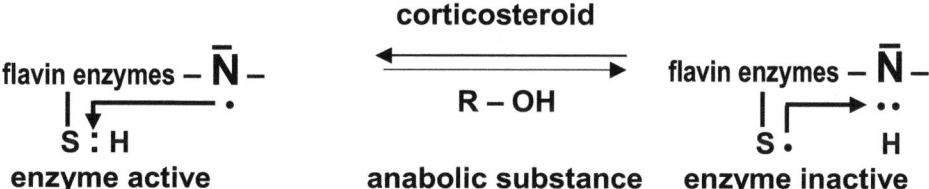

Cortisol → activation of membrane-bound flavin enzymes

Anabolic peptides can only reduce the catabolic activity of the mitochondria by 20% because they cannot reach the radicals inside. The OH group of tyrosine is particularly effective.

Thyroxin → Activation of the respiratory chain by acting as an electron pump to control the flow of electrons and thus ATP for-mation in the respiratory chain. This compensates for reduced O_2 pressure.

There are 2 respiratory chains – in the mitochondria and in the cytosol. The **nucleus** has its own electron transport system.

The latency of thyroid hormones can be reversed by cortisol. Activation of the respiratory chain is only possible with simultaneous stimulation of NADH ubiquinone reductase. However, if this is inhibited, the thyroid is inactivated. This can be achieved, for example, by 6-week protein abstinence.

The *ratio* of the individual components to each other, i.e. the **level of the regulators**, determines the predominant metabolic state (anabolic – catabolic). Different gene areas are activated and thus cause the induction of certain enzymes that are needed for the present metabolic state. The **amount of enzymes** therefore depends on the level of the regulator. This is therefore determined by the *weakest* partner. What prevails is therefore always the result of a *deficiency* (cf. Fig. 22) – a frequently encountered principle.

By sealing the lysosome membrane (lower release of proteases, ribonucleases, etc.) as well as increasing substrate levels, the situation *stabilises.*

Receptors

The mechanistic idea of the docking of certain substances is no longer tenable according to today's knowledge. If receptors were actually present for all substances, the surface of a cell would not be sufficient.
Instead, the receptors are actively built up or broken down by the cells, depending on what the cell needs at the time. An active, intelligent process!
They also contain protein kinases, which is why they themselves can interact with the regulators and a separation for nucleus and cytoplasm is possible (via phosphorylation).

General dephosphorylation immediately reverses the effect, so that it is possible to switch very quickly from anabolic to catabolic and back.

Practical tip:
We know about the problem of adrenal exhaustion in chronic diseases, which can occur after only a few weeks. But if no or too little cortisol is produced, the cell metabolism can no longer normalise because all three components must be present in full.
This is the reason why many asthmatics or rheumatism patients can no longer manage without cortisone.

The same applies to the thyroid gland. Today, it is **not** possible to verify so-called dysthyroidism with the usual examination methods. Unfortunately, the secretion of thyroid hormones that is not adapted to the daily fluctuations does not show up in the blood values because the range of the normal range is too wide. However, we see many such patients in the practice with the typical symptoms of such a disorder. Here, too, it must be assumed that the metabolic regulation cannot take place correctly. Whoever does not take this into account and does not support the endocrine glands in case of insufficiency (organ ampoules, energetic treatment), or substitutes accordingly, cannot expect that the patient will be cured!

Due to the special spatial structure of the receptor molecules, they can resonate with very specific oscillation frequencies, enabling subtle control processes. This is also confirmed by practical experience. The metabolism of a cell can be bioenergetically regulated from the outside by transmitting the necessary information from the regulators. This is easily possible with VEGA-SRT, ZMR 703 and MRT 503. The adjustment takes a maximum of 5 minutes.

This seemingly complicated interaction can be explained very simply using the example of a sphere that is located on a curved plane, exactly at the apex. It remains there if no forces act on it. However, a minimal impulse is sufficient to make it roll (basic regulation through electrons). If it has not yet moved far from the centre, a small force is again sufficient to stop it or to make it roll back to the middle. However, if it has already travelled a further distance (adaptation to strong stress), then it requires greater effort to reach the initial state again. The superordinate hormonal regulators are more strongly stressed (represented by the horizontal arrows).

This is possible up to a certain limit. If this is exceeded (continuous stress), metabolic derailment (anabolic or catabolic) occurs and the disease becomes chronic. This is where outside help is needed. Which one it should be can be seen from the horizontal arrows.

If the metabolism has been permanently shifted to anabolic, then there is a lack (deficiency!) of **catabolic** activity. Patients are conspicuous by chronic fatigue up to and including depression, weak defences, lack of body heat and pasty tissues. They tend to slow down, chronic inflammation, stiffening and hardening (rheumatism, MS, liver cirrhosis).

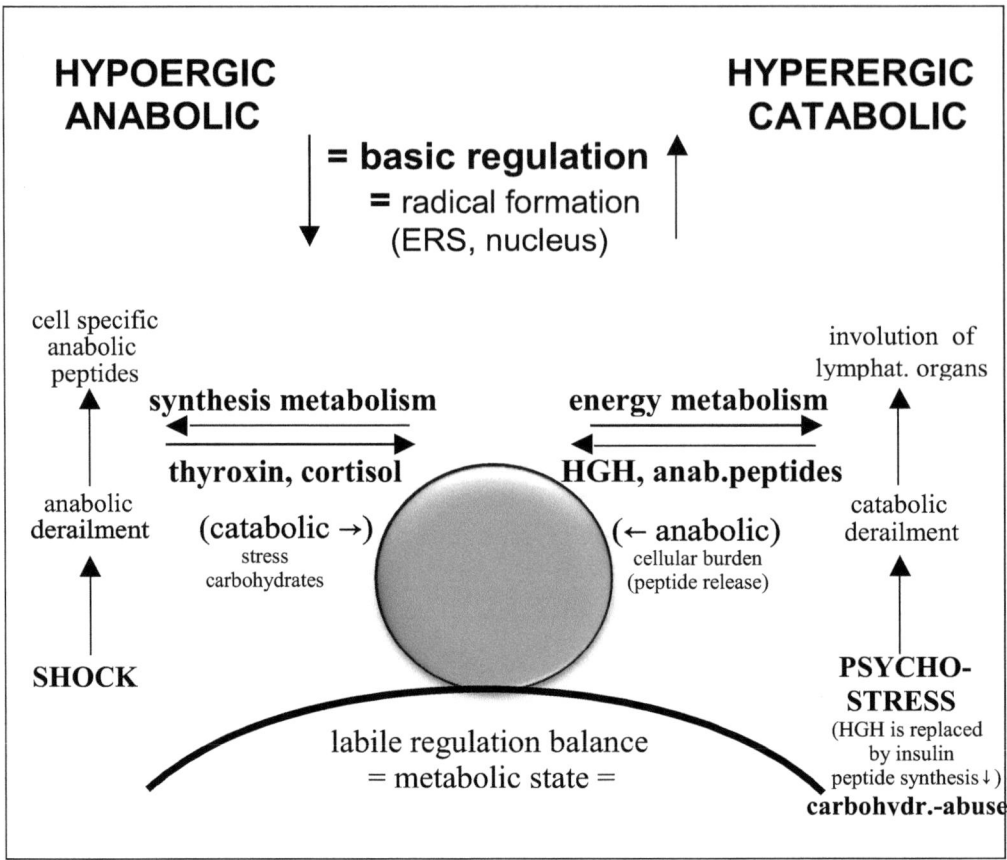

Fig. 19: Basic regulation of cell metabolism and derailments (from "Living Systems Information Therapy", B. Koehler)

Cortisol and thyroid hormones have a *catabolic effect* and can influence the process favorably, but only if cortisol receptors are still present in the nucleus and sufficient HGH can be secreted.

If there is a catabolic metabolic derailment, there is a corresponding lack of **anabolic** activity. The main symptoms are degenerative phenomena (all "-oses") as well as degenerations up to cancer, central heat with peripheral cold (if there is hyperacidity), no reserves, rapid exhaustibility. In addition, there is often forgetfulness and concentration disorders up to dementia.

In both metabolic states, the organism tries to compensate with counter-regulation, which can mask the original symptoms. An anabolic derailment such as a dental granuloma often leads to catabolic symptoms such as cardiac arrhythmia, restlessness, etc. This is why it is always important to consider a focal strain. Therefore, a hidden focus problem should always be considered.

A distinction must be made between catabolic (or anabolic) metabolic states in which regulation is still possible. In children, this includes ADHD, any form of nervousness, lack of concentration, learning difficulties, etc. The growth hormone HGH would help here or the anabolic peptides in the cell, if they are produced sufficiently. However, the release of HGH is usually blocked by two factors – *carbohydrate abuse* and *long-term psychological stress* (see later). But HGH alone would have no effect based on the three-component theory, but only together with cortisol and thyroid hormones, which must be present in sufficient amounts.

The predominantly anabolic metabolic conditions include recurrent inflamemation and the wide spectrum of allergies.

Of the total average of the chronically ill, about 80% have a catabolic metabolic state, mostly as a counter-regulation of a (local) anabolic derailment, which is why the most frequent diseases are found here: From cardiovascular diseases, tumorous degenerations, to ulcerative colitis, Crohn's disease, chron. pyelonephritis etc. Since the primary aim here is to increase anabolic activity via HGH release, this point deserves special interest (cf. Fig. 22).

In addition to the glutathione system and the redox system, there is also the sulphydril disulphide system. The reduction of the sulphur radicals or the mixed disulphides formed from them is possible with an NADPH-dependent glutathione reductase.

Anabolic effects

The anabolic effect of a substance results from the impulse that was able to decrease the radical concentration. This is caused by anabolic effecting substances (initially in the cytosol), which leads to an increase in membrane permeability for sodium, potassium, calcium, as well as an increase in glycolysis and synthesis rate.

Anabolic peptides are radical scavengers and inhibit cortisol-induced catabolism. They are tissue-specific. Their function is supported by

- **fat-soluble vitamins** (including B12)
- **biogenic amines** (serotonin, histamine)
- **prostaglandins, leukotrienes**
- **ginsenosides**
- **heavy metal compounds CuSO4, arsenic**
- **substances with hydroxyl and amino groups**
- **nitriles and nitrogen oxides**

SH-glutathione has a strong anabolic supportive effect.

The formation of fat through the induction of fatty acid synthase (malate enzyme) and alpha-glycerophosphate dehydrogenase by insulin is dependent on T3 and cortisol. Glucagon inhibits this induction.

Specific hormone effects
Adiuretin (vasopressin) has a catabolic effect.
Glucose and glycogen are formed by the interaction of **corticosteroids + insulin** (= anabolic peptide). **Glucagon** only has a supporting function.

HGH + insulin induce the formation of **somatomedins** in the liver, which play a role especially in connective and supporting tissue (cartilage!). As anabolic peptides, they cause the provision of the "fibroblast growth factor" (= second messenger).

Somatostatin inhibits HGH secretion. It is activated by insulin and always increases simultaneously with insulin. It is formed in the hypothalamus, the delta cells of the pancreas and in the intestinal tract and is released in an oscillating manner.

Adrenaline + noradrenaline release T3/T4 very rapidly, via which profound catabolic regulation is possible. One can survive without the sympathetic nervous system, but not without the vagus nerve.
Activation of flavin enzymes and thus cortisone-like effects cause catabolic keto groups.

- **methylxanthines**
- **isopropylaminodihydropyrogallol**

The cortisone-like (only faster) effects of cAMP:

- **rapid increase in glycogenolysis**
- **lipolysis**
- **glconeogenesis**

The "nested" functional principle of metabolic regulation makes it difficult at first glance to make clear statements about the situation at hand in the patient. We have not learned to think in polar terms, which is necessary here. In addition, we have to distinguish not only 2, but actually 12 different metabolic states, because acute processes can overlap chronic ones. Then the symptoms are often not clear. The only thing that helps here is local measurement.

$$\text{metabolic state} = \frac{\text{synthesis metabolism}}{\text{energy metabolism}}$$

But the organism itself does not make it easy either, because both pathways, synthesis (SM) and energy metabolism (EM), have to be managed *side by side* in one cell. This requires the *reducing environment* of the anabolic metabolism, but at the same time the *oxidising environment* of the catabolic metabolism. It is a general problem of the single cell and all multicellular organisms. It can only be solved with spatial separation by membranes.

Anabolic activity takes place in the *cytosol* and is controlled by the nucleus. Catabolic activity is facilitated in the *mitochondria* and is also controlled by the nucleus, although they have their own DNA.

The role of structural fats

At this point, something should be said about structures, because it concerns the cells themselves. In particular, we are concerned here with the role of those fatty acids that do not float around freely in the tissue, but are

incorporated into cell membranes and fulfil important tasks there. Unfortunately, the importance of the *highly dynamic* fat metabolism is completely underestimated. We should ask ourselves why so many structures of the organism consist directly of fat or its derivatives. Fat is known to be an excellent energy store (cf. Chapter 2). The special thing about fat, however, is that it is very reactive and can be metabolised particularly easily, through various pathways.

On this occasion, *cell membranes* must also be attributed a more complex *function* than is generally the case. Their complicated structure can only be understood in terms of the dynamics with which they fulfil such diverse tasks. Unfortunately, their high functionality comes at the expense of stability. This is the real weak point of the cell. If the membrane potential of -70 to -90 mV can no longer be built up, metabolism is no longer possible. Then we are at the end of any regulatory medicine.

Fats are involved in the special membrane structure in a special way. The double lipoid structure is not built by chance from cis-fatty acids (linoleic and linolenic acid). Due to their special spatial arrangement, these fats bind a large number of free charge carriers, the so-called π-electrons (cf. Chapter 2). These have a high affinity to low-frequency sunlight (red spectrum, 630 nm), with which they resonate, which not exactly coincidentally has a high penetration depth into the tissue. These building blocks thus act like "solar batteries", which is a little-noticed feature of the organism.

Linoleic acid is also detectable in many other structures (protoplasm, nerve cells, etc.) and is active as an electron donor to promote vital, energy-consuming processes (in combination with sunlight and oxygen). Above all, they provide energy for the necessary detoxification, including the elimination of heavy metals, and regulate the acid-base balance through their alkaline behaviour. Trans-forms of fats stop these processes, so we can see polar behaviour here again. The cis-form is very unstable because of its reactivity (= autoxydation, reacts immediately with oxygen, among other things) and must therefore, because it is essential, be constantly replaced from the outside. This is promoted by cortisol, but inhibited by oestrogens.

However, the **structural fats** play an important role for another reason: they are a strong insulator, i.e. they can take on a capacitor function by forming a double membrane (not to be confused with the good conductivity of lipoproteins!). In this context, they are of crucial importance for the electrodynamics in our organism. Depending on how they are charged, they form the ground for the vital *potential vortices*. These are induced by move-ment and depend on the conductivity. The worse this is, the more vortices can form.

Due to its affinity to sulphhydryl groups, cis-linoleic acid binds to glutathi-one and cysteine, among others, which is important for cell detoxification. However, during the detoxification and deacidification processes (buffer effect), they themselves are consumed or damaged. Free radicals, heavy metals, toxins and other chemical substances (medicines!), but microwaves and also high-energy radiation (radioactivity, X-rays), even (heated) satu-rated fats (e.g. poly-oils in tinned fish or mayonnaise as well as heated salad oils), or hardened fats in margarine, as well as preservatives, pickled sausage and nitrites destroy these unsaturated fats, resulting in ageing processes and cell degeneration. This change in the environment also provides a breeding ground for a wide variety of parasites.

Local hyperacidity is an unmistakable sign of the depletion of unsaturated fatty acids, but also of free electrons.

The destruction of the fatty acids and the appearance of the unphysiological trans forms creates a new problem. The fats are mostly bound to proteins (lipoproteids), which makes them water-soluble. Other important properties are the stimulation of mucus secretion from the glands and improvement of the flow properties of the blood and thus capillary perfusion. Due to destruction, they clump together and change from liquid to solid form. This results in local stasis with lymphatic congestion or microcirculatory disorders.

A change in the fats themselves due to damaging influences, or the frequent intake of *trans*-forms and other saturated fatty acids favour this. Because of the catabolic metabolic state of the endothelium, these also occur on the inner lining of the vessels and are the precursors of arteriosclerosis (see there). Atheromatous plaques are the typical feature of the stressful solidification of fats (but not colesterol!). At the same time, performance decreases (due to the failure of the "solar battery"). The performance of the immune system is also reduced by the lack of binding to glutathione and cysteine, with all the consequences.

Practical tip:

In order to stop this degeneration process, or even to reverse it, more highly unsaturated fatty acids should be consumed in combination with protein. This is achieved with the oil-protein diet according to Budwig (see under "Nutrition"), which supplies the health-promoting lipoproteins. The experience with all degenerative diseases, including cancer, is excellent, which is why such a diet should not be missing from any dietary recommendation.

The effect is, however, considerably increased with sunlight radiation at the same time. In the cold season, this can be done with special lamps, e.g. red light.

The breakdown of deposits of degenerated fat is supported by enzymes and lactic fermented vegetables.

Everything that has a destructive effect on fats simultaneously paralyses cellular respiration and leads to internal suffocation. This does not always have to be cell death, but can cause the cell to switch from aerobic glycollysis to fermentation. This is what we find in the cancer cell. Otto Warburg already postulated a disturbance in the respiratory chain as a primary cancer characteristic. However, he was still missing an important building block – the highly unsaturated fatty acids.

Vegetative nervous system

Through networking with the **vegetative system**, acetylcholine (anabolic) and noradrenalin (catabolic) have an additional modulating effect. This is particularly evident (catabolic) when there is an increase in *permanent stress factors* (foci, toxins, etc.).

The optimal function of the special control circuits is only guaranteed on the basis of a stable basic regulation.

In practice, this means that in the case of any kind of dysfunction, the metabolic regulation must first be looked at and possibly corrected before going into detail, e.g. to a focal point rehabilitation. Often the problem then solves itself.

Highly interesting interconnections arise with the **sex hormones** – oestradiol (anabolic)/progesterone (catabolic) and testosterol (anabolic)/corticosteroid

(catabolic). Occurring insufficiencies of the endocrine glands (menopause in men or women) have a corresponding effect.

Women (also) differ from men in this respect. She has two hormones that make her more resilient in stressful situations: Cortisol <u>and</u> progesterone.

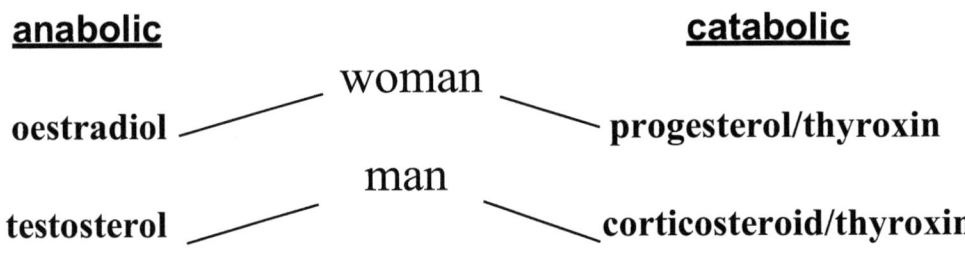

The reason is easy to understand. During pregnancy, oestrogen levels rise sharply, which switches the metabolism to anabolic. In order to provide the necessary energy, catabolic activity via the thyroid and adrenal glands would now also have to be increased. The thyroid gland is (normally) capable of this continuous load, but not the adrenal gland.

In order to spare the adrenal gland, this task is performed by the progesterone. If the woman is not pregnant, she can switch to it in times of high stress and thus spare her adrenal glands.

The polar metabolic regulation has further practical effects. We can very often observe that menopausal women tend to be more overweight and have great difficulty maintaining their weight. Laboratory tests usually show a decrease in progesterone (already from the age of 42!) with still normal oestrogen production, or only a slight reduction. This means that the anabolic hormones predominate with all the consequences – including chronic inflammation. Progesterone can then be very helpful.

Another factor is the organism's constant striving for inner stability. When a woman is exposed to increased stress, which has a catabolic effect, the metabolism increasingly adjusts anabolically to compensate for the deviation from the norm. This opens the scissors. The liver and adipose tissue are highly anabolic, while the rest of the organism is catabolic. This is the same constellation that we find in every pycnician.

If the stressed woman now comes to rest (e.g. at night or at the weekend), anabolic activity predominates and the weight increases.

Now it is also known that HGH, which could bring a predominantly catabolic metabolism (cardiovascular diseases, cancer, etc.) back to normal, cannot be released when the insulin level is high (due to too many carbohydrates), or psycho-durable stress prevails (inhibits HGH-releasing hormone).

The following relationship applies

insulin ↑

carbohydrates
permanent mental stress

HGH ↓

immune deficiency
lack of antibodies

Networking with other hormonal regulatory systems

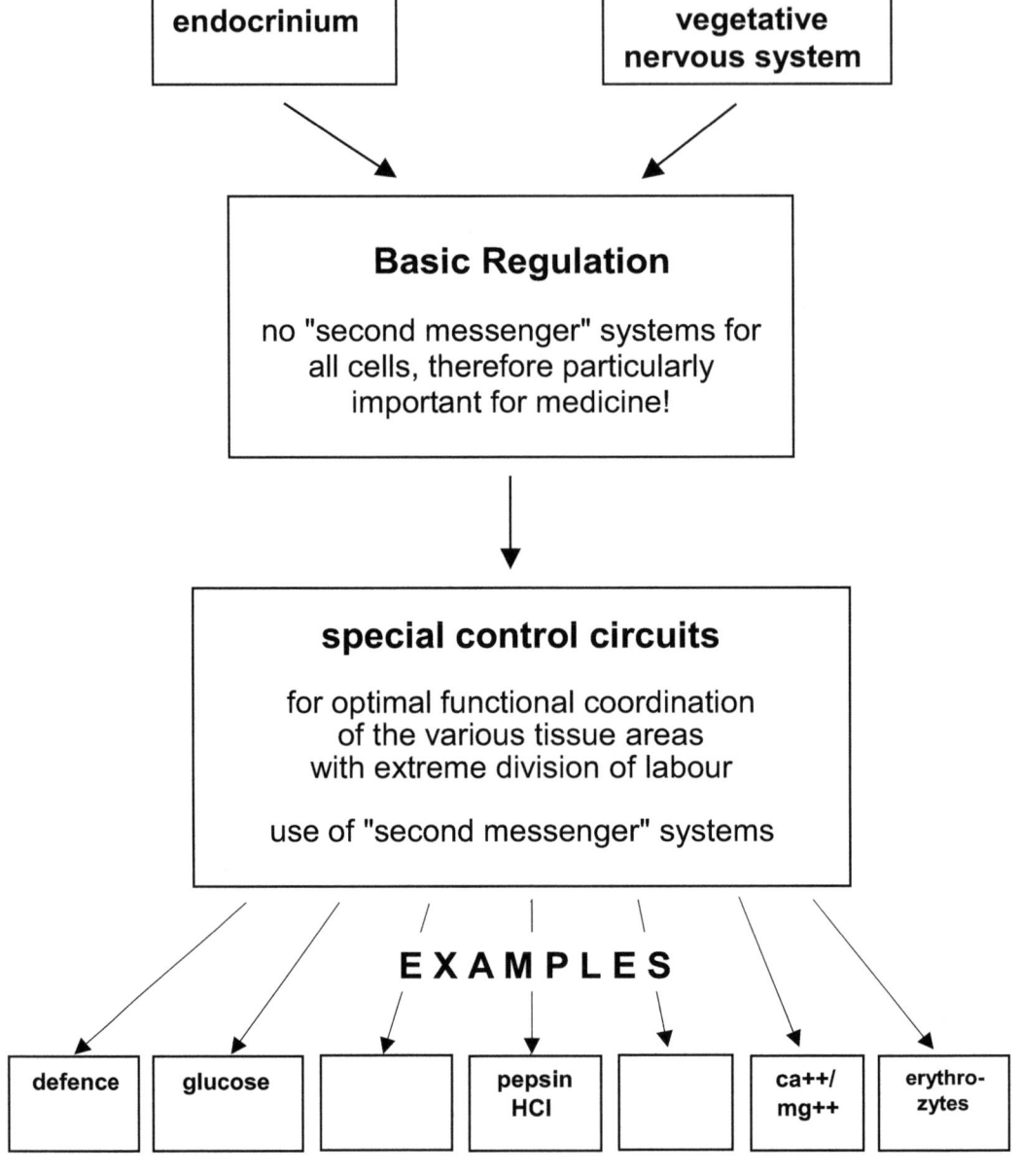

Fig. 20: Differentiation of the basic regulation from the special control circuits

Practical tip:
In a woman with weight problems, the hormone levels should be determined on the 10th and 20th day and the oestrogens (estriol, oestrol and estradiol) should be put in relation to the progesterone. In the case of progesterol deficiency, substitution should be carried out, e.g. with natural hormone from the yam root. Natural oestrogens (also commercially available) come from the pomegranate, among others.

Furthermore, stress should be consistently reduced. This does not only refer to external stress, but also to internal "permanent stress" caused by foci, toxins, etc.

Thirdly, short-chain carbohydrates must be eliminated from the diet because they prevent the release of sufficient STH, which according to the three-component theory is indispensable for normalising cell metabolism.

Regular continuous exercise (not less than ½ hour) leads to fat burning via the muscles.

Since we are dealing with about 80% catabolic metabolic conditions in practice today, it is recommended that all these patients – therapeutically or prophylactically (e.g. stress-ridden managers) – adhere to a strict 6-week *carbohydrate restriction*. This includes potatoes, cooked (!) carrots, industrial sugar, cereals (pasta, bread), rice and maize. After this period, everything can be eaten again, but significantly reduced or replaced by integral products. This causes insulin and somatostatin levels to drop and HGH to rise again. This finally allows the anabolic counter-regulation to get going.

However, there are 3 contraindications (as these are classic *anabolic* derailments: Liver cirrhosis, sarcoidosis and rheumatic forms. Furthermore, it should be noted that severely ill patients should only start the diet under medical supervision, as initially (due to the counter-regulation to HGH) increased cortisol must be released, but this cannot happen with an exhaustted adrenal cortex. This situation should be recognised in time and counteracted by countermeasures (metabolic regulation therapy SRT, ZMR 703, MRT 503). Anabolic peptides can also be administered together with cortisone (low dose, e.g. cortisone D 6 tablets) to help control conversion problems.

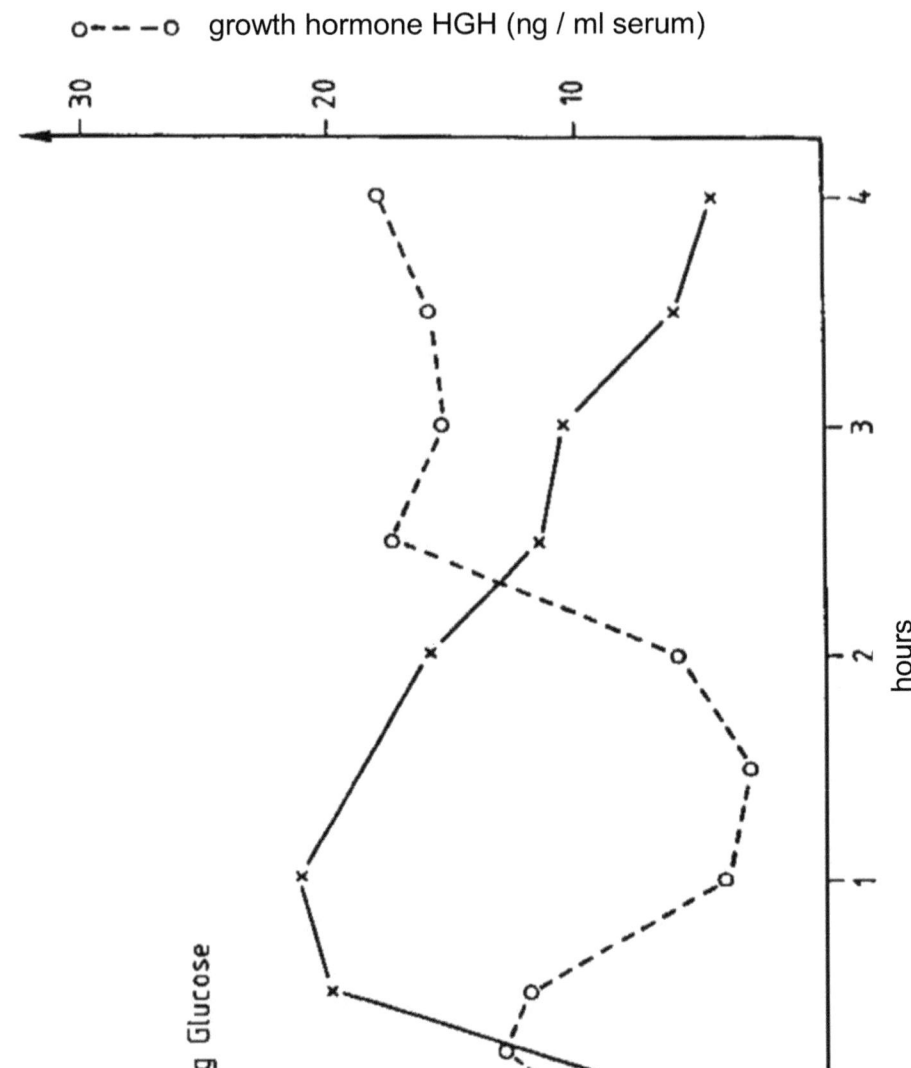

Fig. 21: Influence of the serum level of HGH by the supply of glucose. Both curves – HGH and glucose – are mirror images of each other (from Schole/Lutz "Regulatory Diseases").

The results of this dietary change are usually subjectively felt to be very positive. Blood tests sometimes also show astonishing results. For example, low and high iron levels due to inflammation can normalise. Polyglobulia also responds well.

Elevated triglyceride levels as real heart risk factors drop dramatically, as do blood sugar and insulin. Latent diabetes can normalise under this.

Antibody production decreases, which can normalise autoimmune diseases. At the same time, the risk of cancer decreases and ageing processes slow down, as anabolic regeneration processes are possible again. This also affects the blood vessels, which is why arteriosclerotic changes can be demonstrably reduced and can even dissolve completely.

If the fat intake is increased at the same time as the carbohydrate diet (through Budwig's oil-protein diet), the metabolism often changes after only 4 weeks.

The low-carb diet can also be followed for longer as a health care, age and cancer prophylaxis.

However, as can be seen from Fig. 22, there is a whole range of other factors that can contribute to an inhibition of the balancing component. From this point of view, the reason for a ***failure to heal*** (not the disease itself!) can always be sought in the fact that the ***balancing forces cannot become effective*** for various (!) reasons.

Practical tip:
Here we can clearly see why hyperinsulinism must lead to a chronic immune deficiency. We find this, for example, in children who eat a lot of sweets. You can often recognise them by the fact that they have a constantly running snotty nose. These are the so-called lymphatics.
But diabetics are also included here, because often it is not the exhaustion of the pancreas that is the cause, but an insulin resistance with increased blood sugar levels.
Children who have growth problems (HGH deficiency!) should be fed only very cautiously with carbohydrates. In the case of the others, who shoot up uncontrollably, the increased intake would have a slowing effect. The targeted use of nutrition can therefore control the growth in length, but the associated normalisation of the metabolism can also reduce the susceptibility to infections that is usually associated with this.

Health lies exactly in the middle between anabolic and catabolic, whereby an oscillation around this middle value results from circadian rhythms. The characteristics of a chronic illness show themselves in a loss of rhythmicity (through which, according to H. Heine, homeostasis is established), as well as the impossibility of coming into balance on one's own. It can therefore be classified as *anabolic* or *catabolic*, depending on which part predominates.

Unfortunately, the names are misleading. Actually, diseases should be named according to where the deficiency lies, because that is also where therapeutic action must be taken. The assignment "anabolic" means that this condition is predominant (e.g. bronchial asthma) and tempts to use an "anti" drug. However, the blockage is on the catabolic side and should primarily be solved there *by support!*

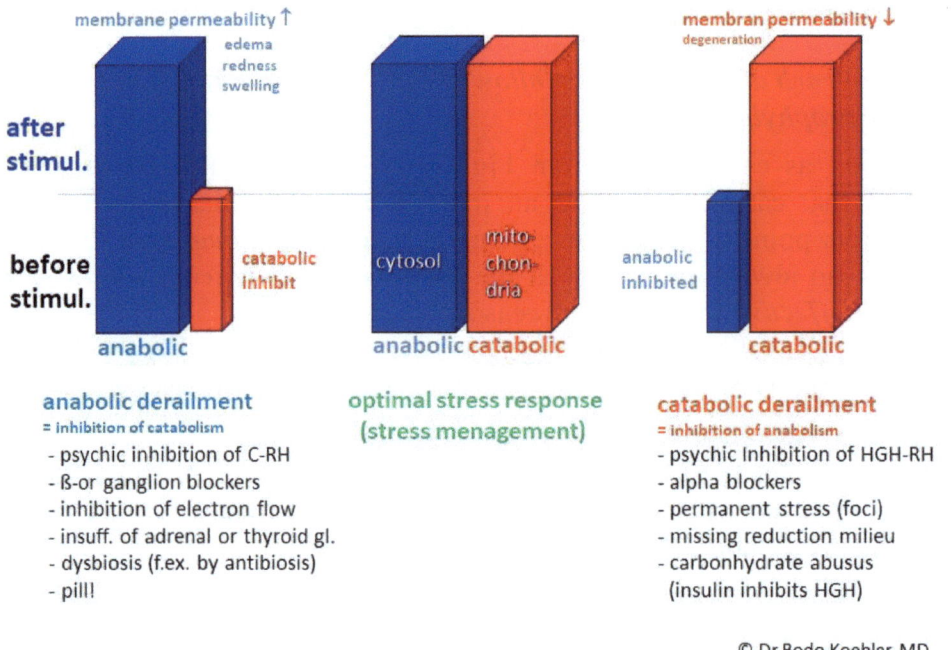

© Dr Bodo Koehler, MD

Fig. 22: Metabolic regulation and insufficient load adaptation, left of the catabolic, right of the anabolic limb (from "Cancer – a cureable disease", B. Koehler, Bod-Verlag).

> **Practical tip:**
> The effect of alpha-blockers, for example, should be taken into account here. They inhibit anabolic activity and thus promote catabolism. However, they are recommended in cases of high blood pressure, for example, a catabolic disorder, which completely prevents normal metabolic balance.
>
> On the anabolic side (e.g. in rheumatism, asthma, etc.), the situation is similar with the prescription of antibiotics. By destroying the intestinal flora, any healing process is suppressed because the catabolic metabolism is blocked. In both cases, psychological stress prevents the release of regulators. In the case of anabolic diseases it is the cortisol, in the other case the HGH-releasing hormone. Co-treatment of the psyche, also through phytotherapy or Bach flowers, is therefore absolutely necessary.

Electrolytes

Research into the basic regulatory system by A. Pischinger have shown that four main electrolytes (Sod., Pot., Ca, Mg) are of particular importance as they influence the polar stimulus-response behaviour of the matrix. The adminis-tration of individual fractions therefore has a direct effect on metabolic regulation. Sodium and magnesium have an anabolic effect, potassium and calcium a catabolic one. This is the reason why magnesium is used with the same success in (catabolic) heart diseases as calcium is used in (anabolic) *acute* allergy.

> **Practical tip:**
> When prescribing the orthomolecular preparations that are so popular today, more attention should be paid to the ratio in which the 4 main minerals are contained. If sodium and potassium, or calcium and magnesium are balanced, they behave neutrally, i.e. they will not change the metabolism. However, if a metabolic effect is desired, which is usually the case with chronic diseases, then the mixture should be changed accordingly.
> This is of particular relevance for catabolic cancer, because here (catabolic) calcium administration is absolutely forbidden.

Minerals

Deliberately, a distinction should be made here between electrolytes and minerals. We know a total of 81 elements (3^4), which are arranged in the periodic system according to a system of 7 (4 +3). But 4 of them form a kind of platform (compare 4 elements), and are directly interrelated with each other.

The 4 main minerals sod. – pot., as well as mg – ca are in a polar relationship to each other, but are again interconnected, because they also obey the law of four. At the latest since the matrix research by Pischinger,

but certainly from experience already much earlier it is known that they exert a decisive influence on the stimulus-response behaviour of the matrix in addition to the fibrocyte charge and the hormone pattern present at the time. Of course, this also refers here to the switch anabolic – catabolic.

Stimuli can deepen or fix a certain metabolic state, but also lead to a reversal. If a catabolic metabolic state is present, then a strong anabolic stimulus can be set by targeted movement, but also by tapping massage, and as a result a healing reaction can be initiated.
All other elements also play a role in the organism, which is usually only noticed when a deficiency occurs (compare selenium and cancer). It is therefore by no means of secondary importance if *all* elements were actually classified in the Luescher cube, as in this way orthomolecular medicine could be upgraded from a new aspect. Many combination preparations would then have to be reconsidered, but also free combinations could be considered with more scientific background, which of the elements is the 81st and would therefore have a very special significance because it falls out of the system. It could be, for example, that it has a kind of control function.

A completely new aspect is now crystallising through the research of K. Meyl, because the **conductivity** of the tissue depends on its composition of minerals. This is of great importance because the rolling-in and rolling-out processes of the potential vortices depend directly on it.

When we talk about conductivity, we are again talking about the free flow of electrons in the tissue. They are charged with photons (or arise from them in the first place), which have been programmed with more and more experience in the course of life. They form the electron tori, which in their totality are called **bioplasm** (the CHI of the Chinese).

This makes it clear that knowledge of electrodynamics is necessary to approach life processes with the right approach. In medical school, this is only a marginal topic. This deficit should definitely be filled by every inquisitive therapist!

So there is still a lot of work to be done. We are just at a hopeful new beginning.

Optimal *relation* and *sufficient level* of the regulators enable an *optimal metabolic situation* (optimal redox potential in the cytosol, in the mitochondria and in the cell nucleus).

Because of the complexity of the interrelationships and their eminent importance, the *summarising remarks* of J. Schole are reproduced here verbatim: "Building on the Pasteur effect, as the most elementary regulatory principle, all experimental facts and all indications speak for the fact that the **basic regulation** in all cells of a higher organism takes place via the **redox potentiall**, supplemented by the possibilities of **interconversion** and **allostery**.

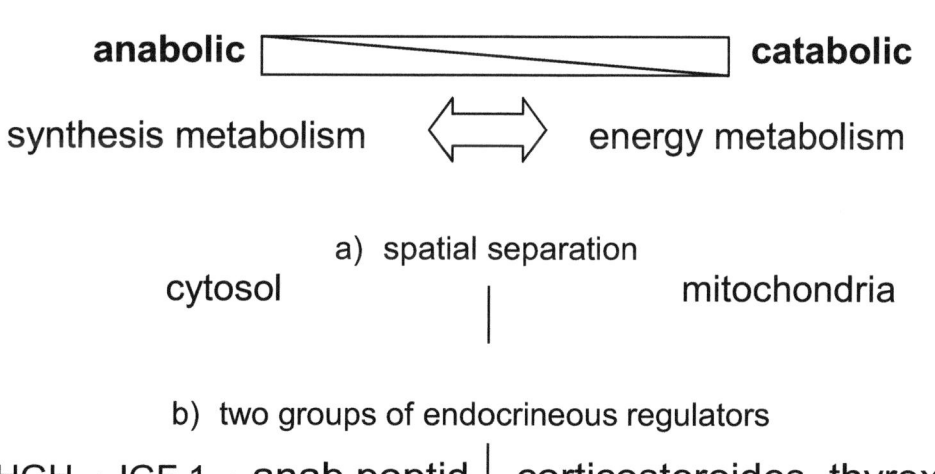

Problem solving in the higher organism:
Adjustment of the respective redox potential
through polar regulatory behaviour.

anabolic ⬚ **catabolic**

synthesis metabolism ⟺ energy metabolism

a) spatial separation

cytosol | mitochondria

b) two groups of endocrineous regulators

HGH → IGF 1 → anab.peptid. | corticosteroides, thyroxin

c) two nervous regulators

parasympath. → acetylcholine | noradrenaline ← sympathicus

Fig. 23: Optimal adjustment of the redox potential by 3 systems

The **"second-messenger systems"** are not used for basic regulation, but for very fast reactions, e.g. in special control circuits, whereby the entire regulatory system experiences close networking. The basic regulation is carried out by **three-component systems:** corticosteroids and thyroid hormones regulate the energy metabolism (in the mitochondria and cell nucleus) as **catabolic components** and peptides provided by somatotropin regulate the synthesis metabolism in the area of the cytosol and cell nucleus (**3 main metabolic hormones of the endocrine system**) as **anabolic components.**

A second system, which – closely linked to the endocrine – is used to *modulate* this basic regulation, consists of noradrenaline as the **catabolic** and acetylcholine as the **anabolic** component **(vegetative).** The components of both systems must be present in the cells in optimal relation to each other at sufficient levels to guarantee an optimal and sufficiently stable steady state between energy and synthesis metabolism and thus an ideal redox status for the various cell compartments (**optimal – stable "metabolic situation"**; corresponds to the term "health").

During **positive stress adaptation**, the main metabolic hormones are made available from the depots within one hour, with a highly significant increase in the functional capacity of the organism. In the case of prolonged stress, an adaptation of the enzyme patterns, mitochondrial numbers etc. to the new situation takes place with the participation of the cell nucleus.

In the case of preferential provision of one component, **regulatory derailments** occur, which have become known as regulatory diseases (**negative stress adaptation;** corresponds to the term **"chronic disease"**). In the case of strong mental stress, the provision of somatotropin is disturbed ("adaptation syndrome"), in the case of shock the provision of corticoids. In between, there are all transitions for all tissue areas.

Knowledge of the concentration and thus the efficacy of both endocrine and both vegetative components in an organism is therefore of extraordinary importance in medicine for diagnostics, therapy and prophylaxis." (end of quote)

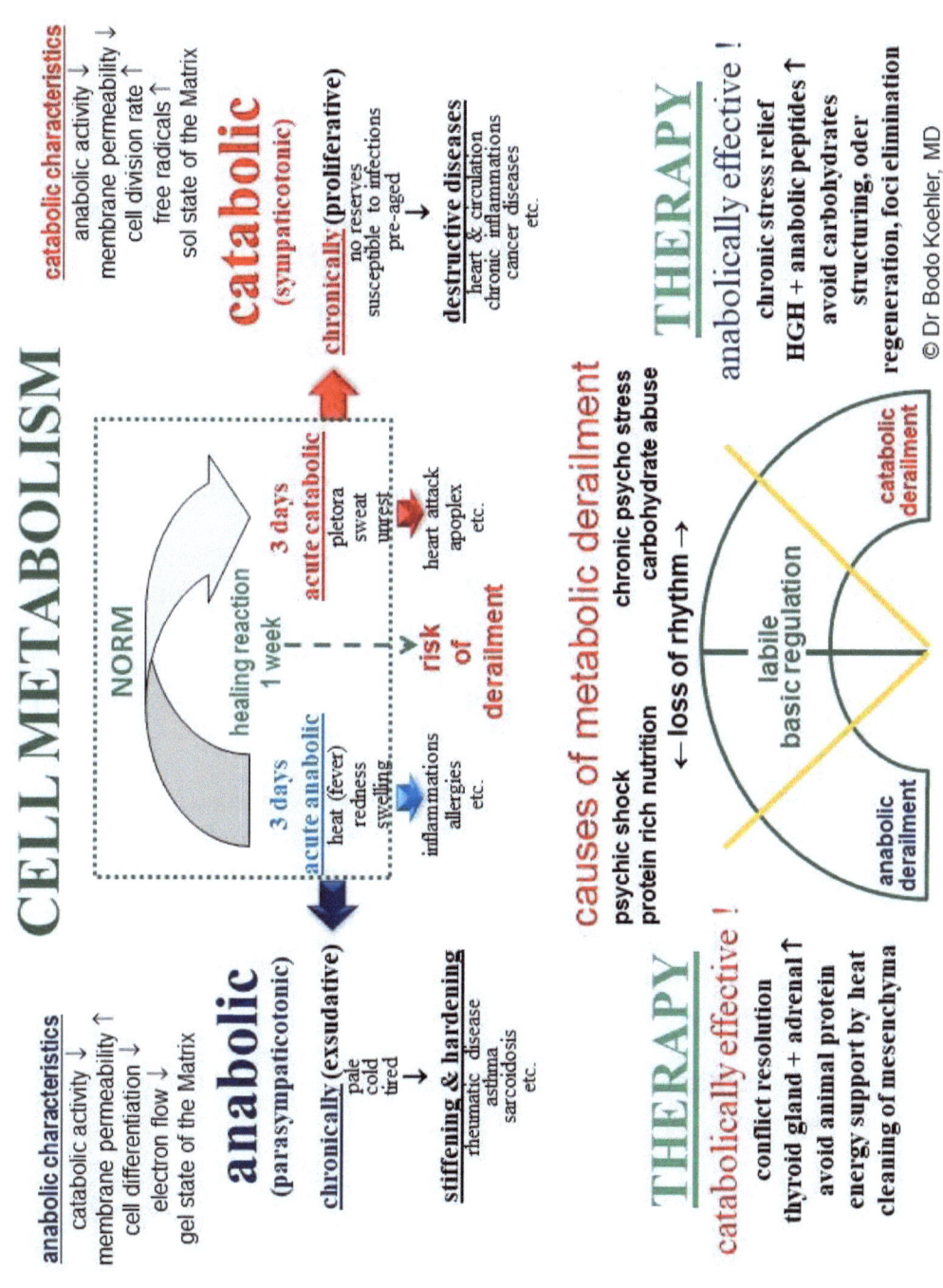

Fig. 24: Metabolic regulation and chronic states

Ways of adapting to stimuli (adaptation)

The organism uses 2 ways to adapt to external stress. One is extremely effective because the total time to complete **stress adaptation** is only 1 hour. However, this only works if the hormone stores in the adrenal gland are full and there are sufficient anabolic peptides in the cells. Unfortunately, we encounter this health potential less and less often. Then even bacteria or viruses could be fought off without the appearance of symptoms. The aim should therefore always be to have full stores, but this cannot be achieved by rest, but only by alternating load and unload, i.e. rhythm.

Acute illnesses *only occur when the cortisol stores or anabolic peptides are exhausted by stress*, because *stress adaptation* is then no longer possible after the immediate reaction (duration 1 hour). In this case, "stage 2" of the defence programme takes place, the alarm reaction according to Selye, which lasts 7 days. The symptoms that occur here (fever, sweating etc.) must be understood as a *healing reaction* and must not be suppressed.

The second path is accompanied by the appearance of acute symptoms and must be understood as a healing reaction so that the organism can rid itself of its invaders in this way. This proceeds according to the scheme of Fig. 18, the alarm reaction according to Selye. Here, the production of anabolic peptides on the one hand and cortisol on the other must first be ramped up before the metabolism can be optimally regulated.

Nevertheless, this pathway is also a physiological variant. Anyone who uses allopathics to suppress fever or antibiotics here has not only misunderstood the principle, but is also doing lasting harm to their patients. The time rhythm is forcibly interrupted and free adjustment around the midpoint is prevented. The consequences are rigid metabolic states, either anabolic or catabolic, without the ability to adapt quickly to changing environmental conditions.

The 2 phases differ not only in time, but also in the different activity of the metabolic states at the beginning.

In the *fast phase*, there is primarily increased *catabolic* activity, which is accompanied by sympathicotonia; in the *delayed* phase, there is primarily increased *anabolic* activity, which is accompanied by parasympathicotonia.

All acute illnesses as we know them follow this pattern (cf. Fig. 19 page 84).

Metabolic Adaptation

fast phase
(asymptomatic)

delayed phase
(acute healing reaction)

- emptying the
corticoid depots
= 30 minutes

- increasing the
corticoid and
peptide production

- release of
anabolic peptides
by HGH
= 60 Minuten

- fast rise of
peptides in the
cells

- optimal
regulator level
after 4 - 5 days

positive
stress adaptation

positive
stress adaptation

Fig. 25: The two physiological pathways of metabolic adaptation

In the literature, one sometimes finds misleading information. However, this is due to the interpretation of the measurement results. Of course, we also find anabolic activity in a catabolic sympathicotonic phase, because metabolic regulation runs according to polar laws. However, what is decisive for the symptoms (not for the therapy!) is what predominates.
Therpeutically we support the deficiency.

> **Practical tip:**
> The organism can react to any stimulus with the fast or the delayed phase. But the difference is almost 1 week! In the first case, nothing is felt, in the second case, acute symptoms appears.
>
> The goal should therefore be to react only with the fast phase if possible. This is achieved by filling up the hormone stores. However, this is not to be achieved by rest (lazing around), but by interval training. This can be done on all levels – from psyche to nutrition to sport.
>
> This would achieve real prevention on a scientific background (cf. "Life-Rhythm-Therapy").

Shock always initially produces an anabolic reaction, such as in shock lung or shock kidney. This is characterised by a flooding of the tissue with fluid because the membrane permeability is increased. This is why cortisone is used in acute care, which stops the influx. This is known to have a catabolic effect, which is why observation in practice once again shows the correctness of the three-component theory according to J. Schole.

One special feature should be mentioned here. When the organism adapts to a stimulus, the metabolic balance takes place at a *higher level*. This means that a higher resilience to subsequent stimuli has been achieved. This is also the reason why sport (in moderation) increases the defence performance.

> **Practical tip:**
> If major interventions are planned for the patient, the resistance can be increased beforehand through positive stress adaptation, which significantly improves the chances of recovery. This is especially important for critical interventions.
>
> This can be done, for example, through Kneipp treatments, or through one-time intensive physical exertion.
>
> In very weakened patients, however, an injection of 50 to 100 mg of cortisone can be administered i.v. 1 hour before (for example, because of an unavoidable surgical intervention). This increases resistance and thus considerably reduces the risk of surgery.

Reset mechanisms

The highly equipped "apparatus" must also regress in an orderly manner after a stimulus in order to maintain economy. This happens in the first phase exactly on the eighth day, after the counter-shock phase according to Selye (cf. fig. 18 page 83) has ended. Then a rapid decrease in corticosteroids takes place, as well as the degradation of the corticoid receptors at the cell nucleus. At the same time, peptide synthesis is repressed. This is followed by a short anabolic phase.

There is a risk of relapse here!

Noxe
⇓
positive stress adaptation
⇓
short anabolic phase
⇓
re-adaptation

Practical tip:

There are many patients who go through a largely normal alarm reaction according to Selye during acute illnesses. Then, however, a relapse occurs. Sometimes even several. Metabolic measurements always show a persistence in the normally short anabolic phase, which is symptomatically expressed in weakness and fatigue.

In these cases, catabolic activity should be promoted with appropriate measures – from sweat baths to a high-carbohydrate vegetarian diet, or directly with metabolic therapy devices (VEGA-SRT, ZMR 703, MRT 503). Preventive action, however, can be taken much more elegantly by carrying out a therapy with the above-mentioned devices exactly on the eighth day (at the latest on the ninth), with the setting "anabolic" (which should of course be tested), in order to support catabolic activity in this way.

Metabolic blockages

The reasons are manifold, but very often caused iatrogenically. Antirheumatic drugs and antibiotics lead to an anabolic, the other "anti's" to a catabolic metabolic derailment and prevent normal regulation (cf. Fig. 22 page 96). The pill is also one of them.

This does not mean that such a procedure should be totally rejected. It only depends on what is intended. But if such means are used without attempting to treat causally, this cannot be approved of. Unfortunately, it must be assumed today that about 60% of all chronic diseases are caused by such interventions.

When states of exhaustion in the cellular metabolic system have occurred due to disease, we often find

- **imbalances in the enzyme systems**
- **substrate deficiency** (also a problem of the matrix)
- **malfunction of membrane permeability** (lipoid structure!)
- **lack of μ-electrons of the lipoproteids**
- **allosteric effects of metabolites** (feedback)
- **inhibition of regulators** (by psyche or insulin)
- **disturbed relation of polar electrolytes**

Metabolic derailments

Every chronification of a disease is caused by the ***inability of the cells to regulate***. The reasons are always of a complex nature, even if apparently only 1 agent is in the foreground. Since we are dealing with a complex networked living system, constitutional peculiarities, external influences, rhythms and daily fluctuations are also involved. But there is always an overload of one or more systems due to one-sidedness. This must be seen as an act of the psyche, because we alone determine how we shape our lives. Even if pressure comes from outside, we always have the choice to go our own way, without external determination. This can lead to tensions, but we should not avoid them in order to remain ***authentic.***

The metabolic derailments can develop insidiously over years, or suddenly. The criteria are shown in the following diagram.

anabolic derailment	catabolic derailment
syntheses run slower	oxydation and radical formation ↑
delayed cell division	frequent cell division
cell size ↑	cell size ↓
epi- & endothelium become thicker	epi- & endothelium become thinner
basal membrane ↑	basal membrane ↓

malfunctioning of the cells

The skin can be used to study how cells shift into a catabolic derailment (degeneration). The thin skin of old age, but also patients who have constantly used ointments containing cortisone, show these phenomena.

Chronic diseases can arise at the *cellular level* due to
- **insufficient repression of peptide synthesis**
- **too rapid decrease in corticosteroids** (after the alarm reaction)
- **too rapid degradation of the corticoid receptors at the nucleus** (cortisol can no longer enter the nucleus)

J. Schole defines *regulation diseases* as follows: "Disproportion between the necessary metabolic state in a certain stress situation and the regulation that actually takes place."

He distinguishes 2 types:

→ **Type I:** Relative deficiency of anabolic or catabolic regulators. The surplus corresponds to the metabolic situation. This results in
- **anabolic inflammatory**
- **anabolic inflammatory proliferative** (when resting tissues are stimulated to grow). This can lead to secondary auto-immune processes
- **catabolic inflammatory** (e.g. intestinal diseases). This can also lead to secondary autoimmunity. Trigger very often psychostress.

→ Type II: HGH is replaced by insulin.

All anabolic diseases have substance-related causes (receptor deficiency) or arise from regulator depletion (adrenal cortex). They tend primarily towards autoimmunity, catabolic ones towards paraimmunity. Antibody formation is an anabolic process, but phagocytosis is catabolic (pollutant removal, viruses, bacteria, fungi).

Allergies and autoimmunity intensify anabolic derailments up to shock (anaphylaxis). Shock conditions occur primarily in tissues with a low reproducetion rate (lungs, kidneys).

All diseases *are divided into anabolic and catabolic* because of their symptoms. In each case, however, the cause is the failure of polar metabolic activity (energy or synthetic metabolism). The underlying blockage must be diagnosed and specifically treated. It can lie on *all levels of existence*, from the psyche to deeply material.

Every chronic disease should therefore primarily be examined to determine what has disturbed the normal metabolic regulation. The first step is to determine the current metabolic state (local and overall).

Already in the fifties, Heilmeier and co-workers had carried out measurements on patients and found allocations. A summary of these results is shown in Fig. 26.

Those diseases that are not listed can be classified on the basis of their symptoms. Carcinoma, for example, is also missing. It clearly belongs to the catabolic diseases, whereas lymphomas are anabolic.

The classification is made easier by further criteria:

anabolic	catabolic
order	chaos
cold	heat
fever (acute)	sweating
alkaline (acute)	acidic (infarcts)
acidic (foci)	alkaline (distribution)
inflammatory exudative	inflammatory proliferative
oedema formation	degeneration
membrane permeability ↑	membrane permeability ↓
cell differentiation	cell devision

Tissues that are highly dependent on HGH are epi- and endothelia, connective and supporting tissue, and the defence system. These are particularly at risk for catabolic derailments.

Further information can be found in the learning aids, chapter 8.

It should be noted that certain organ diseases occur twice, but with different faces. Glomerulonephritis is anabolic (increased permeability), pyelonephritis is catabolic. It is similar with ventricular ulcer. The anabolic ulcer would heal under cortisone administration; the catabolic one would break through. This alone shows how essential knowledge of the metabolic situation is for the correct assessment of the patient in practice.

Figure 26 must not be understood in such a way that the listed diseases (the illustration goes back to Heilmeyer) would always be found in the area shown. This only applies to the "resting state". These patients cannot reach the normal position of zero, which would mean an even activity from anabolic to catabolic of 50% each, because either the anabolic or the catabolic metabolism cannot reach full activity.

But when strong stimuli hit, the system has to react. It will, however, behave in a way that corresponds to its possibilities. This means that an anabolic patient will become even more anabolic, a catabolic one even more catabolic.

Furthermore, it must be taken into account that an otherwise healthy person can also (temporarily) reach these metabolic states. However, the decisive factor is that the latter is in a metabolic dynamic, whereas the chronically ill patient is in a state of rigidity.

Therefore, metabolic measurements should always be taken before and after stimuli in order to reliably distinguish rigidity from a transitory state. For this purpose, a stimulus is set after the first measurement and a measurement is taken one minute later. This was already realised two decades ago with VEGA-SRT (metabolic regulation therapy) and further developed in ZMR 703 (cell & milieu revitalisation). A completely new variant was realised in MORAnova device. It is based on these presented scientific principles.

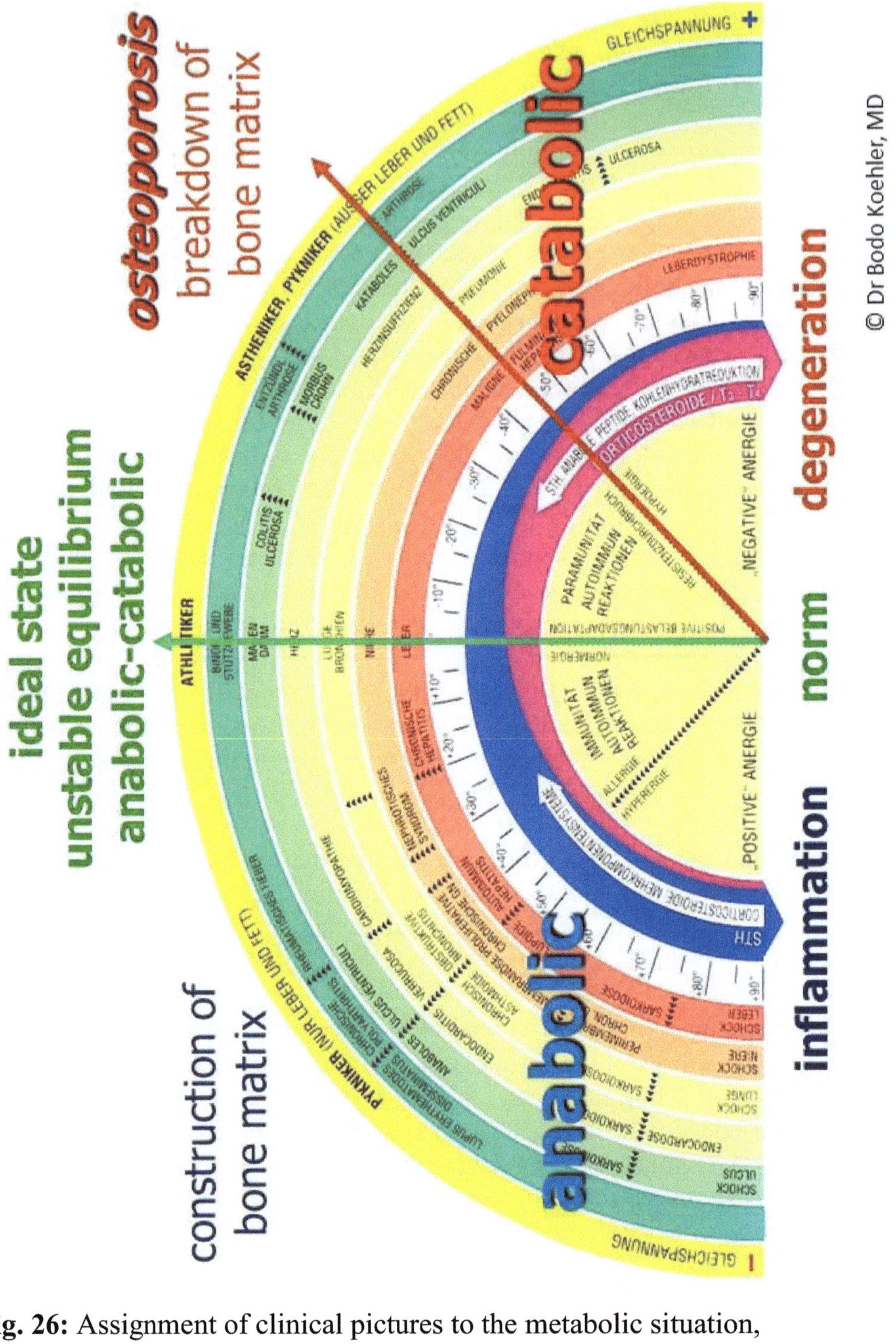

Fig. 26: Assignment of clinical pictures to the metabolic situation, especially in case of osteoporosis

If metabolic measurements are repeated at certain intervals, the progression curve gives an even clearer picture of the regulatory behaviour and the individual dynamics. This is particularly valuable for assessing the efficiency of a treatment regime.

Diseases of civilisation

Many of the diseases have to do with our lifestyle, with lack of exercise, wrong eating habits, psychostress, etc. The degree of stress can be seen in the *altered metabolic regulation*. This makes it possible to give clear guidelines for treatment that have an exact scientific basis. At the same time, inconsistencies can be uncovered that arise in therapy or diet recommenddations if *no* reference is made to the laws of metabolic regulation.

Arteriosclerosis *is caused by a catabolic metabolic derailment of the endothelium, due to excessive consumption of carbohydrates, with simultaneous energy-consuming anabolism of liver and fatty tissue.* The cholesterol level and the blood fat level (triglycerides) do not play the primary role! No atheromatous plaques can develop without the catabolic (acidic) metabolism (due to lack of anabolism). The increase in neutral fats is the *result* of constant carbohydrate abuse, not the other way round.

A causal treatment in this case is therefore also carbohydrate restriction – and not fat renunciation – with simultaneous reduction of psychodurable stress. Only in this way can the progressive degeneration of the blood vessels be stopped and regeneration (!) initiated. Highly unsaturated fats (omega 3) have a supporting effect in combination with protein as *lipoproteids*. Glucosamine and vitamin K2 can also be used (e.g. Glukosa-K2®). Endurance sport is also advisable (has an anabolic effect).

Cholesterol *is our most important vital factor and is built up to 80% by the organism itself (liver, brain). It is a component of all cell membranes and offers protection during inflammation.* Then it is increasingly synthesised. Cholesterol is not a fat, but a steroid and thus the starting material for all important hormones (including cortisol) and must be produced in greater quantities under stress (catabolic metabolic state). The chronic increase in cholesterol is a stress parameter – not a risk factor! It can indicate chronic inflammation foci. The medicinal reduction of an acquired hypercholesterolaemia without clarification of the internal or external permanent stress causes must be classified as malpractice. Cholesterol has nothing to do with the development of arteriosclerosis! In USA, studies were carried out according to which a *lowered* cholesterol level (below 180mg%) resulted in an increased risk of cancer.

J. Schole says: "Under civilisation conditions with a high-carbohydrate diet, the cholesterol level can only be used as an indicator of the high-risk metabolic state of *energy-consuming anabolism*, which leads to catabolic counter-regulation."

So if it is considered that the reason is the chronic catabolic stress metabolism situation, which "gives us" the civilisation diseases because of the blocked anabolic activity, then everything should be done to increase the total anabolic activity (GAA). Fig. 27 shows what is helpful in this. This should be studied carefully for this purpose.

Increasing the "Total Anabolic Activity (TAA)" of the serum by different pre-treatment
(glutathion-state test; rats; male; weight: 177-277 g)

pre-treatment	application	time (days)	increasing the "Total Anabolic Activity" of the serum %
zero control	-	-	-
NaCl	0.1 ml/day i. p.	5	100
		10	150
HGH[1]	100 µg/kg/day; 0.1 ml i.p.	5	3900
		10	7900
germination control	-	-	3900
running training[2] without ginseng	-	28	300
running with ginseng	125 mg/kg fodder	28	900
carbohydrate restriction (isoenergetic)	15% fat[3]	28	400
	30% fat	28	4900

[1] bovine HGH   [2] once a week until exhaustion   [3] tallow/lard 1 : 1

SCHOLE et al., J. Anim. Physiol. a. Anim. Nutr. 71, 156 - 168 (1994)
SZÁSZ und SCHOLE, unveröffentlicht (1989)
SCHOLE und LUTZ, Regulationskrankheiten, Enke-Verlag, Stuttgart (1988)

Abb. 27: Feeding trials with and without fat content to increase total anabolic activity (from Schole/Lutz "Regulation Diseases", BoD-Verlag).

The surprise is perfect when the figures are compared that result from carbohydrate restriction in animals. It is shown here that the combination with *low-fat* feeding (after all) 400 % increase was achieved. However, if the fat content was doubled, then a 4900 % increase can be recorded!

These experimentally obtained findings can be considered a sensation, as they make a mockery of most dietary recommendations, which advise abstaining from fat in catabolic diseases. If *fat consumption* is advised here, this can of course be further specified. Attention should be paid to a high proportion of unsaturated omega-3 fatty acids, which should best be ingested in an oil-protein compound.

Osteoporosis is also a catabolic, degenerative condition. Therapeutic efforts should therefore go in a similar direction, namely to increase anabolic activity and avoid catabolic mechanisms. A key role in this is played by a testosterone deficiency.

This example shows how wrong, even damaging, the official opinion is when calcium intake is recommended. Calcium has a catabolic effect and therefore aggravates the condition. Magnesium, the antagonist would be correct. Besides, the *skeleton* of the bones (that is what breaks down) is 75% silica and sulphur, not calcium. The latter is only stored for consolidation.
Daily silica supplements (e.g. Sikapur, KlinSiMag® or similar) have been shown to increase bone density. Furthermore, as with other chronic degenerative diseases, reduction of psychostress, endurance training and the intake of highly unsaturated fatty acids in combination with protein as well as magnesium also apply here.

The calcium recommendation for osteoporosis must be considered particularly devastating because it can activate a latent cancer. A cancer patient should always avoid increased calcium intake! Possibly the increase of breast cancer in the population has a real cause here.

Gout is not a rheumatic disease, as is unfortunately sometimes claimed. It is a degenerative condition and can be understood as a *catabolic form of gluconeogenesis* through muscle breakdown (!). The main thing is to avoid carbohydrates; only secondarily do the purine bodies play a role.

Since in the meantime we also have to add the patients who have been damaged by allopathic treatment (approx. 500,000 per year in Germany alone!) to the civilisation ailments, a few references to this should also not be missing. Antibiotics and antirheumatics (always!) cause an anabolic, most of the other allopathics a catabolic metabolic derailment. This is the mechanism of action when treatment is not causal but only symptom suppressive.

In summary, 4 causes can be identified for the diseases of civilisation:
- **carbohydrate abuse**
- **psychological stress**
- **lack of exercise**
- **destruction of lipoproteids** (entropy)

If we consider that 2/3 of all diseases affect the cardiovascular system and are degenerative diseases that cause immeasurable damage to the national economy and devour many billions, then we should really make every effort to find a remedy. If we also consider that the causes are now known and therefore causal treatment or prevention can actually take place, then it is absolutely incomprehensible that this knowledge is not consistently implemented. Instead, pseudo-wisdom is spread, for example, that bacteria (chlamydia) are possible causes, because then, of course, appropriate antibiotics can be sold. Bacteria or viruses only ever play the role of the trigger that causes specific symptoms (of the defence reaction!), but are never causa.

In times of Corona, this misconception, which goes back to Robert Koch, became a billion-dollar grave. Those who *actually* died of Corona were comparable to the annual flu deaths. But the sums of money spent for vaccinations with unclear effects were astronomical.

However, I do not give up hope that common sense and the truth will prevail for the good of all. In this case, that would mean that first of all there would have to be a worldwide clarification from official agencies that clearly points out cause and effect, with corresponding approaches for successful treatment.

Depending on the stage, the following measures should be taken more or less consistently. This would not only be favourable for avoiding the degenerative diseases of civilisation, but also chronic inflammations, up to and including cancer. This could mobilise an enormous health potential!

Basic recommendations for diseases of civilisation

1) **Balancing stress loads through regular breaks**
2) **Drastic reduction of sugar-like carbohydrates**
3) **Avoidance of heated or hydrogenated oils and artificial Trans fats**
4) **Intake of lipoproteids** (oil-protein diet, see later)
5) **High-quality protein from organic farmers**
6) **Intake of lactic fermented vegetable juices** (up to 1 l daily)
7) **No kitchen stress with appliances (loss of electrons!)**
8) **Start with light endurance training** (1/2 hour daily)
9) **Take magnesium supplements while avoiding (!) calcium, possibly zinc and iodine (both are often lacking).**
10) **Sufficient sun exposure to charge the lipoproteins, but do not use creams with a protective factor.**

This does not say everything (e.g. avoidance of noise), but the direction is marked by these sensibly coordinated components. If these 10 points were followed even approximately, millions of people could be helped immediately.

If you want to pamper yourself additionally, you can listen to good classical music, but not with headphones, but through loudspeakers at a normal volume (like at a concert), so that the vibrations can be felt physically. In this simple way, the degree of order in the tissues is significantly raised. Certain therapy methods have this as their goal. Techno music or other rhythms produced with synthesisers cause rigidity in the organism and thus weaken the health potential (cf. Chapter 2).

All these measures are at the same time the necessary *basis* for 80% of chronic diseases, on which further therapeutic measures are built, which can thus achieve much more success. At the same time, this activates the cooperation of the patients and thus improves compliance. Many patients expect specific rules of conduct from their doctor and are grateful for every hint.

The more a patient is sensitive to cold, or possibly also electrosensitive, the more he is overacidified, which is an unmistakable sign of a lack of lipoproteids (LP) and thus free electrons. LPs have a deacidifying effect by binding the acidic H^+ ions to them. However, this destroys them themselves and they fall out – if there is a lack of free electrons. These micro fat clumps can cause circulatory problems, which is why the enzymes and lactic acid products should be used to remedy the situation.

Nowadays, the increasingly popular mobile phones present our organism with a new, hardly manageable problem of information chaos. Those who believe they cannot do without them should at least use a hands-free device (earplugs) or an external antenna and refrain from using the telephone in closed rooms and cars.

Smoking is also known to have an unfavourable effect. It increases the catabolic metabolism in the vascular system and additionally promotes arteriosclerosis, apart from the carcinogen benzpyrene. Smokers inhale about 10^{11} free radicals per breath! Therefore, abstainers should not spend too much time in the vicinity of smokers.

Immune system

When the function of the immune system is to be assessed today, the so-called immune status is usually used, a count of the cell numbers. This is comparable to a barracks, where the number of soldiers is determined – but nothing is noted about the equipment, training level and condition of the soldiers. The *function* of the defence cells, antibody production and mobility are inextricably linked to their cell metabolism, which brings us back to the topic.

The stressed person is only more susceptible to infection because his anabolic metabolism is blocked. HGH is the strongest immune-stimulating hormone we know.

Immune system and metabolic regulation belong together and should be understood in their interactions.

In the case of immune deficiency and chronic consumptive diseases, all inhibiting influences on the release of HGH should be avoided. These include permanent psychological stress as well as the consumption of too many carbohydrates. The production of antibodies is an anabolic process, whereas phagocytosis and thus all detoxification processes are catabolic.

An important partner of the defence system is the redox system, in conjunction with the glutathione system. Both work independently of each other, but are often involved together. Here, radical processes play a major role, just as they do in the basic regulation of cell metabolism, as does the sufficient supply of cis-fatty acids.

The **redox status** alone determines metabolic activity:
- more oxidation >>> more catabolism in the mitochondria
>>> less synthesis in cytosol and nucleus
- more reduction >>> more anaboly in cytosol and nucleus
>>> less catabolism in the mitochondria

The **cell nucleus** is subject to a 4-phase periodicity that controls cell division. Two anabolic and two catabolic phases can be distinguished.

Radicals *must be considered in a differentiated manner*. They have a destructive effect preferably in catabolic metabolic *derailments* and should only then be defused with radical scavengers. Anabolic diseases show a lack of free charge carriers, which is why radicals can be very helpful here. Radical scavengers should therefore only be used very cautiously and judiciously in catabolic disorders.

Practical tip:
Due to the absence of free radicals and excess of electrons (reducing environment) in anabolic diseases such as rheumatism or asthma, for example, ozone therapy (ozone is a 2nd order radical), or singlet oxygen (1st order radical) can be used with great success in the context of HOT.
The situation is different in catabolic diseases, which are characterised by an excess of free radicals. Here, ozone should only be used under the protection of antioxidants. HOT, however, can be used for both metabolic conditions because of its scavenger function.

Measurement methods of metabolic regulation
It certainly does not require much explanation to understand that the highly dynamic metabolic processes cannot be adequately recorded statically. Only through frequent measurements, or after provocation, can a useful statement be made.

What is important?
The diagnosis is based on the organism's inability to regain balance on its own. It is therefore a matter of detecting blockages. It is not enough to determine the metabolic situation, but the cause should also be determined – on all levels of being – which has led to a deviation from the norm. As already mentioned, this can be of many different natures. However, it is important to discover the characteristic that has interrupted the *dynamic* of being, the ability and willingness to change.

In doing so, we always come back to mental processes, which have the strongest influence on our organism and represent the actual driving force. Under no circumstances, however, should the material aspect be neglected. Spirit, soul *and* body must always be brought into harmony. On a physical level, the *energy balance* is the indicator of well-being, which is reflected in the body heat.

The measurement methods commonly used today come from functional medicine. Fine-energy test procedures are used such as Vegatest, BFD, electro-acupuncture, kinesiology, etc., in connection with metabolic devices such as VEGA-SRT, ZMR 703 or MORA*nova*. With this, the current metabolic situation can be determined, which always simultaneously gives indications of the organic problem (with organ-related measurement), or of the loss of vital information (with meridian-related measurement), but *at the same time* of the underlying psychological cause. This enables the therapist to support an expansion of the patient's consciousness through targeted discussions, in which the categorical ordering system, the Luescher cube, is particularly useful.

In order to put metabolic regulation on a scientific basis, objective blood tests are necessary. However, not all parameters are suitable for this. Ultimately, the decisive factor is the determination of the "Total Anabolic Activity" TAA. However, since not all anabolic peptides are known yet, this is a difficult task. The HGH level, which could be used as a reference, fluctuates too much and is therefore not reliable. IGF-1, or better still IGF-3, provide a more accurate statement. There is still a lot of development work to be done for the discovery of further anabolic peptides. In the future, however, it can be expected that such analytical methods will be available.

Individual tissue peptides can be determined via HPLC (high-pressure liquid chromatography). This would make it possible to determine metabolic disorders of individual organs or to recognise the effect of diets or forms of treatment (therapy effectiveness!). At the same time, a prognosis would be possible, as overloading of certain organs could be detected at an early stage.

Another possibility would be to determine the degree of inhibition of membrane-bound flavin enzymes. An in vitro test would be suitable for this, in which the L-amino acid oxidase would be inhibited by anabolically active substances. It is found in the outer mitochondrial membrane.

For the sake of completeness, the ***glutathione status test*** acc. Schole should be mentioned, in which the radicals are inhibited in vivo. However, this is not possible without puncturing the organ.

In the meantime, the pyrexal test according to Heilmeyer (1964) has historical value. This is a real functional test in which the breakdown of wheals is observed, which disappear at different rates after Pyrexal injection depending on the metabolic state.

Energetic procedures are still the method of choice because they lead to immediate results, which is indispensable in practice. However, to substantiate these results, and of course also for quality control, blood tests could be carried out in parallel, whereby an objective proof procedure for the effect of certain forms of therapy up to and including medication would also be possible.

Conclusion

All these findings about metabolic regulation, which have been presented here in fast motion, lead to the following ***core statements***, which form the basis for the daily work with patients:

1. **every change in the internal or external conditions must be compensated for by the open system "human being" by adaptation under energy consumption – ENERGY BALANCE.**

2. **the necessary metabolic regulation is only possible if the 3 components HGH, cortisol and Thyroxin are present at the same time – REGULATORS.**

3. **the metabolism works according to polar laws. The anabolic and the catabolic metabolism are activated simultaneously, with different WEIGHTING.**

4. **every chronic illness indicates that this mechanism no longer functions and that the metabolism can no longer be adapted due to blockages – DISEASE.**

5. **symptoms always express the deficiency. It is the deficit in the attempt to compensate for a one-sided load. This is where the loss of RHYTHMIC shows itself.**

6. **inhibiting factors which prevent the metabolic balance and a normal load adaptation are to be sought on 3 levels: PSYCHOLOGY, NUTRITION, IATROGEN.**

Without the primary restoration of metabolic normalisation, healing is not possible. For this it is necessary to create the conditions for energy absorption (photon absorption) through nutrition and to eliminate the stresses on the matrix on a morphological level in order to increase the degree of order.

Summary of metabolic regulation

All chronic diseases can be divided into two groups: One with rigid anabolic metabolism (due to decreased catabolic activity), the other with rigid catabolic metabolism (due to decreased anabolic activity). The goal of therapy must be to support the weaker area, regardless of the level at which the patient is approached. This applies to psychotherapy as well as to dietary counselling, medicinal or energetic treatments. Thus empiricism becomes causal, life-supporting medicine.

Without knowledge of metabolic regulation, which was explicitly described by J. Schole in his three-component theory, pathophysiological processes in the organism cannot be correctly assigned, resulting in misinterpretations.

Both anabolic and catabolic activity is always present at the same time, because the polar principle also applies here. In the resting state, both are equally strong, which is guaranteed by the basic regulation.

In order to achieve an adaptation of the metabolic state, all 3 components (T3, T4 and cortisol for catabolic, HGH or anabolic peptides for anabolic) must be present simultaneously in the cell and cell nucleus.

Adaptation to strong stimuli (infections, trauma at all levels) depends on the initial state, i.e. the hormone stores. In a rested state, adaptation occurs within 1 hour. Under stress, it takes 1 week and is associated with the appearance of acute symptoms. Nevertheless, this can still be considered physiological (healing reaction).

Only the chronic disease indicates the derailment of the metabolism, which has arisen due to the deficiency of one part (anabolic/catabolic). This is where the therapy must start. Not the predominant part is fought, but the deficiency is balanced by strengthening the weaker part. To do this, different levels must be taken into consideration.

work scheme
metabolic state

measurement
symptom
kind of disease

SM 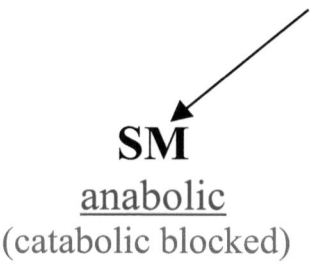 **EM**

anabolic   catabolic
(catabolic blocked)   (anabolic blocked)

levels

SM	level	EM
liver and fat tissue	←localisation→	rest organism
Pycnics	←phenotype→	Asthenics, Pycnics
cortisol↓, T3,T4↓	←regulators→	HGH↓, f.e. insulin↑
coppled	←information levels→	decoppled
permeability↑	←membranes→	permeability↓
size↑, amount↓	←cells→	amount↑, size↓
gel state	←matrix→	sol state
right brain switched off	←hemispheres→	left brain switched off
head left↓	←kinesiol. test→	head right↓
shock	←psyche→	permanent stress
proteins no	←nutrition→	carbohydrates no
gymnastics	←exercise→	active movement
cold improves	←temperature→	heat improves
↕	(only if acute – otherwise vice versa!)	↕
blue	←colours→	red
no	←scavencher→	yes
ca/pot./cu↓	←minerals→	sod./mg/zn↓
progesterol↓	←hormones→	oestrog./testost.↓
constitutions therapy	←LSIT→	perm. stress relief

Regulation, however, is only possible if there is sufficient energy (heat balance as an indicator) as well as life information. These universal properties are carried by the photons. The material basis for this is formed by the highly unsaturated fatty acids in combination with proteins and oxygen. These should be adequately supported through nutrition, as should the removal of used fats.

6. Nutrition

Awareness of nutritional issues is still far underdeveloped – among the population as well as among therapists. The reason for this certainly lies in the cherished habits that need to be abandoned. Yet food is the basis for survival, in the constant confrontation with the most diverse stresses.

"Diets" always have the flavour of sickness and restriction. But there is another way: correct nutrition increases the joy of life, improves the dynamics, increases the defence, promotes regeneration, raises the mental well-being and has a balancing effect in stress situations. To achieve this, however, some cherished ideas about the intake of material ingredients (vitamins, minerals) as the only effective components of food must be thoroughly revised.

The first surprise usually follows when it is made clear that our food cannot cover the actual energy needs of the cells. We also need additional a lot of ambient energy, which we get directly or indirectly (e.g. oven heat) from sunlight. For this, however, certain prerequisites must be present, which we in turn must create for ourselves through our diet. This includes, among other things, the sufficient supply of highly unsaturated fatty acids (cf. chapter 2), but also the intake of *information and order*, which is contained in every food. This is usually completely overlooked. Animal protein is difficult to digest, but it contains very complex information and a high degree of order, which is necessary for the organism. It therefore has a strong anabolic effect, but cannot be considered a comparable energy source to the easily digestible carbohydrates or fats.

The food itself usually contains sufficient energy for the digestion process. The ratio is clearly surplus in the case of carbohydrates, and approximately balanced in the case of protein. Excess calories are consumed immediately, or radiated as heat. This would give us a balanced diet without getting fat or losing weight. The frequently observed weight gain in the population is usually not due to a calorie surplus (except in the case of frequent eaters, others deliberately eat little but gain weight anyway), but to the type of preparation – hot or cold (often lacking the necessary heat of combustion) as well as to an inappropriate composition (too many carbohydrates in a sedentary lifestyle), which then shifts the metabolism to the anabolic side.

Additional aspects must be integrated into the nutritional recommendation, such as individuality and constitution, modalities such as place, time, climate, situation, age, type of preparation, mood, as well as polar inter-actions.

In order to be able to consider the manifold effects, an overarching theo-retical concept is needed, which is offered to us by the three-component theory of metabolic regulation by J. Schole, in connection with the well-founded, millennia-old knowledge of the Chinese about the flow of the life energy Qi.

The polar consideration of anabolic and catabolic food (or YIN and YANG) provides a new understanding of healthy nutrition and nutrition that supports the healing process. Rhythm plays an important role here. Through the frequent alternation of stress and relief, the health potential is gradually raised through nutrition and thus a healing process is intensively supported. This releases vitality, which Hippocrates had already postulated.

Every form of nutritional intake has a direct effect on the regulation of the metabolism and thus on the course of disease. Its importance can there-fore not be overestimated.

First of all, however, a strict division must be made between a sick diet and a health-maintaining diet. It is completely absurd for a healthy person to follow a certain diet. One should eat a varied and wholesome diet (according to Kollath). It can be useful to separate proteins from carbohydrates in order to facilitate digestion (cf. Hay). But here, too, the main rule is

Eat with joy and pleasure, pay attention to the ambience and good mood.

Any diet that is doggedly followed does more harm than good! A diabetic who eats an ice cream sundae with great relish has done more for his health than the neighbour who denies himself this "sin".

If Hippocrates was right that our food should also be our remedy, then there must be something wrong with the current nutritional teachings. Diets some-times have a supporting effect, but as we know and use them, they do not have a healing effect on serious illnesses. The reason is probably that our "western" nutritional guidelines are characterised by substance thinking, because natural science (what a misleading name!) cannot explain the phenomenon of "life". The living is eliminated by the reductionist approach.

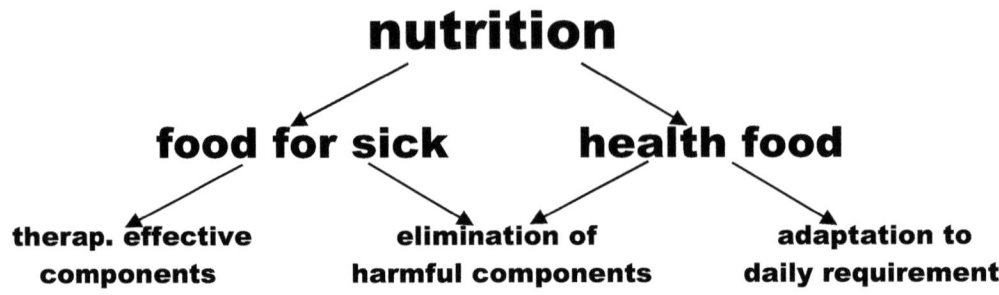

In contrast to this is the "Eastern" approach, which is based on life energy, the Qi. In more modern terms, one can speak of *information* that regulates life processes.

Certainly it is correct to say that certain substances are supplied with food. However, the crucial question is whether the substance as such is important, or whether it is not rather only a *carrier medium*, a kind of preserve for the "message" it contains, namely the *information* transmitted with it, which has far-reaching effects, ultimately on every cell, but also on the psyche, since the two are inseparably connected.

That is why the assessment of the *quality* of a food also appears in a completely different light. F. A. Popp already carried out investigations on food and measured completely different radiation of biophotons, depending on the source and producer. The higher the biological quality of the food, the higher the photon content.

From a scientific point of view, it looks like the electron systems of the "real" food must be in the iso-energetic point to the photons of the sunlight (cf. Spin of the electrons, Fig. 2). The necessary conditions for this were researched by L. Pauling. For example, azo compounds (benzpyrene in

cigarette smoke), silver, anthraquinone, paraffins, polymerised (heated) oils, saltpetre in sausage and preservative radioactive rays have a disturbing effect.

Certain seed oils have π-π-electron systems that are exactly at resonance. The resonance frequencies of sunlight can be calculated with the Schroedinger equation.

Today, therefore, a completely different aspect plays the main role in the assessment of recommendable foods. Meat is not problematic for health because protein burdens the connective tissue (cf. Wendt). This is true in principle, because the free SH groups of some proteins (sulphydryl groups) can have a sclerosing effect on tissue structures. However, this only happens if, due to a lack of unsaturated fats, no water-soluble lipoproteids (association of the proteins with the fats) can form, which not only have a "defusing" effect, but also deacidify.

The only compensating factor for the sclerosing (material compacting) SH-group of the proteins are the unsaturated fatty acids.

In direct dependence on rearing (fattening, animal meal, preservatives fed, antibiotics, livestock farming), meat today often contains more polluting saturated fats in solid form than high-quality (liquid) unsaturated fatty acids, which are the decisive criterion for the quality of a food. Thus, meat is automatically depleted of photon-charged pi-electrons.

The quality of olive oil, for example, can be increased considerably if 1/5 linseed oil is added in relation to the total quantity.

The metabolic state *at the time of food intake* is the basis for all observations. After all, the effects can always be read there. For this purpose, the polar behaviour of the anabolic part to the catabolic (and vice versa) should be observed (cf. Fig. 18, page 80). The effect of a food on the organism cannot be assessed without taking into account the current metabolic situation; it can even be completely contrary! This results in a great many interactions that should be examined more closely.

What are the problem points? In the following, some aspects are listed that have so far either not been considered at all or only insignificantly in the various diets. However, since there are obvious interactions here, this would be a first approach to a new understanding of nutrition.

What are the problem points? The following is a list of some aspects that up to now have either had no significance at all or only an insignificant significance in the various diets. However, since there are immense interactions here, this would be a first approach to the new understanding of nutrition.

Dietary recommendation

The term "diet" is used differently today than the meaning of the word actually implies. Diet should have an *ordering effect* on the organism, which is beneficial every day. It would therefore be completely natural to constantly pay attention to one's diet, to one's order. In Western usage, however, diet is always associated with problems (illnesses, overweight) and thus receives a negative touch.

However, in order to return to the old, positive sense, we will speak of *dietary advice* in the following, in order to create awareness for a completely natural approach to nutrition, to awaken a joyful feeling for harmony and balance, which are solely in our hands and can be controlled by ourselves.

Usually a diet is primarily there to support an organism that is out of balance by restoring healthy order. Classical, rigid diets for prevention or health maintenance should therefore not exist at all, because this can lead to one-sidedness. However, if everyone decides for themselves what to choose from the wide range of culinary possibilities and avoids others, this has nothing to do with a diet in the conventional sense, but much more with flexibility and the very personal situation in which they find themselves at the moment.

A *dietary recommendation* should serve to optimise the functioning of the organism, which can immediately be seen in physical well-being, a balanced mental mood, accompanied by a positive aura. This immediately creates the motivation to continue on this path – in contrast to strict diets (compare diabetes), which only mean renunciation and can thoroughly spoil the patient's joy of life.

If something has to be done without, an equally attractive alternative is needed. This can consist of eating "forbidden" foods and reducing the excess carbohydrates with appropriate exercise.

One-sided diets

Today we are almost dogmatically stuck in various directions. Vegetaria-nism is elevated to the status of a religion by some people – their users feel correspondingly privileged – even though very many of them are more ill than healthy. However, the goal cannot be one-sidedness, but only variety and versatility. To achieve this, various interactions must be included in the consideration, as discussed below. In this way, it is achieved that every person can in principle eat everything, but always at the right time.

However, this does not yet take effect with the start of a dietary change. The organism usually needs 6 weeks to permanently change its metabolism. Therefore, a clear signal should always be given to the organism at the beginning, but only for a maximum of 6 weeks (e.g. strict avoidance of carbohydrates).

Acid-base balance

Acidosis is often hyped up as the cause of diseases, although it is only one – albeit very important – symptom of the disturbed respiratory chain. There, the highly unsaturated fatty acids play an important mediating role. However, one should bear in mind that the common deacidifiers do not address the cause. On the contrary – if a section of tissue in the organism is over-acidified, e.g. in the case of chronic inflammation, then neighbouring areas are compensatorily highly alkaline. A general deacidification could then cause problems in the previously healthy areas and drive them into completely different co-diseases (e.g. rheumatic pain with cancer), which could be avoided if the metabolic situation was known.

Disease-related diets

Only a few people have noticed so far that the individuality (including constitution) of a person is completely ignored by assigning diets to disease patterns. However, this is precisely the domain of naturopathy!
Everyone has the experience of different courses of the same disease in different people. So it is logical that a certain diet must have different effects on different patients.

This is where a very thorough rethink is needed. The goal can only be to develop a very special, very personal *dietary recommendation* for each patient. What almost seems like utopia here is, however, quite practicable, because all the partial aspects listed here can be traced back to a common, unifying basic principle.

Climate

Anyone who goes on holiday to a hot country experiences very drastically what influence climatic characteristics have on nutrition and well-being. It makes a big difference whether I eat the same meal on a cold or a very hot day. Since the metabolism is programmed completely differently, the results are correspondingly different. On a hot day, the catabolic energy metabolism is drastically reduced, which results in general sluggishness, but in a positive sense in stress reduction and relaxation. People tend to reach for cooling drinks or drink a lot and eat only light salads. Every heavy meal is instinctively avoided or regulated by the lack of hunger. These are general experiences that can be used therapeutically.

Cancer shows a strong catabolic activity. External heat reduces this (compare hyperthermia). All "fast burners" (certain carbohydrates) should be avoided, as otherwise the catabolic metabolism would be activated (at the same time there would be a blockade of the HGH release via the increase in insulin, see Fig. 21 page 95). All foods that promote *anabolic* metabolism are therefore recommended. This includes above all meat and other proteins. Accordingly, on cold days, internal heat should be stimulated, as some foods otherwise lead very quickly to weight gain. Even a hot soup as a starter can be very helpful and prevent this, but the preparation of the food itself is also essential.

Preparation

Whether a food is taken cold or hot, whether it is raw or cooked, fresh or seasoned, juicy or dry, whether it comes from the greenhouse or from the field, etc., has very different effects. Special attention should be paid to the preparation, because the effects on the metabolism can be drastically different.

The importance of the intact molecular structure of food is emphasised below in "Structure and Order". Water also has an internal structure (cluster domains) and can therefore store information. In the tissue it is present in crystalline-liquid form (H. Heine). The worst thing that can be expected of food is to defrost frozen food in the microwave.

However, another point is rarely considered, and that is the free electron content of a *food* (!), which is responsible for its freshness and therapeutic benefits. By processing vegetables or fruit (smoothies!) with motor-driven devices, almost all electrons are sucked out by the magnetic field of the motor, making the product worthless or even harmful to health. The usually

negative redox potential then reverses; it becomes positive and the fruit or vegetable becomes an electron robber!

Combinations

The 4 (!) main groups in nutrition **protein, carbohydrates, fat** and **water** are not metabolised in parallel, but influence each other. If, for example, fat is eaten alone, it is immediately converted into energy, causing the tri-glyceride level in the blood to drop. However, if carbohydrates are present, they are first converted into energy, which promotes a peripheral catabolic metabolism, with simultaneous anabolism of liver and adipose tissue (see Fig. 27 page 113). Therefore, it is not fat per se that is the cause of arterio-sclerosis, but the combination with carbohydrates. Primarily, carbohydrates should be reduced, especially white flour products.

Fats

Again and again one reads that fats should only be used very sparingly, without, however, mentioning in one word which fats are involved. It is true that all hydrogenated (margarine!) and heated oils should be avoided, the more consistently the better. The reason, however, is not the danger of increasing cholesterol, because it does not occur in fat at all (as it is a steroid), but the destruction of lipid structures and the precipitation of degeneration-promoting solid fats, which are no longer able to absorb photons and act as energy stores (cf. Chapter 2). They are only a burden for the organism, as they lead to microcirculation disorders and local lympho-stasis.

Enzymes are needed to dissolve these deposits. The intake of lactic fermen-ted vegetables is helpful.

Location

Everyone has certainly had the experience abroad that some food tastes excellent locally – including the wine, but the same ingredients can almost arouse disgust at home. These geographical peculiarities are related to the soil, the sunlight and, last but not least, the geomancy – the natural health-promoting field of the earth. A general recommendation is therefore to eat local food as much as possible, also in relation to the season. In this way we stabilise our body field. Fruits or other exotic products must always be understood as stimulus meals. This can sometimes be quite helpful because it forces the body to regulate, which can mean regeneration. For an ailing organism, however, it is stress.

Exercise

A person at rest, e.g. during sedentary work, has a completely different metabolism than under physical stress. High-performance athletes, e.g.

runners, therefore have a different diet than heavy athletes. The different stresses of the day also require an adapted diet. The intake of carbohydrates in particular should be made dependent on this. The more exercise, the higher the proportion may be. Of course, this also applies vice versa. Other factors, e.g. periods of high stress, must also be taken into account when *recommending nutrition*. Therefore, food intake should be planned in advance in order to be fit for the coming events. In this way, reserves are conserved.

Mental mood

Eating can and should be fun. Through a successful meal, we can build up a high potential of positive energy, which stimulates us mentally and in this way helps us to move forward. Sometimes it is not so much the meal itself, but the ambience and the good mood that sets in. *Quality of life* is the keyword that should be included in any *dietary recommendation*. This includes a lot of variety and trying out new compositions, even from foreign countries. Life is about drawing from the abundance on offer.

Age

The diet of a baby and an old person can be very similar. Both eat porridge. But that is not what is meant here. A child's metabolism is designed for growth, so high anabolic activity combined with high catabolic metabolic activity. The old person shows predominantly catabolic activity because anabolism is reduced. This results in degenerative diseases. Therefore, the diet should primarily be oriented towards whether it can increase *anabolic* activity. At the same time, increased attention should be paid to internal heat (from page 150).

Water

The greatest attention should be paid to the No. 1 food, namely water. This applies first of all to drinks. The supply of minerals (missing or in excess) has a direct effect on the metabolism. The ratio of potassium to sodium plays just as important a role as the quotient of calcium to magnesium. It is also important to consider whether the drinks are taken before, with or after a meal, whether they are hot or cold, acidic or alkaline, and so on. Depending on this, they promote or reduce catabolic metabolic activity.

The other aspect is the water content of the food. The more water they contain, the more they have a cooling effect, which lowers catabolic activity and thus promotes weight gain. However, if such foods are heated (e.g.

tomatoes), then this effect is cancelled out and even reversed. Anabolic, water-containing foods then have a strong catabolic effect.

Rhythm

Life is rhythm. The homeostasis of the tissue is established through rhythms (H. Heine). Just as a regulated sleep-wake rhythm serves to maintain health, we have an excellent opportunity to intervene very directly in the body's rhythms in a simple way with nutrition. This special approach should apply to the day, the week, the month and the year. In the case of serious illnesses, healing processes can be triggered by rhythm alone. Taking into account the Arndt-Schulz rule, supporting and inhibiting foods are recommended in alternation. In this way, the regulatory levels can be forced and the health reserves increased (cf. Life-Rhythm-Therapy).

Structure and order

If the molecular lattice structure has been destroyed by external treatment (loss of order), an essential part of food has lost its meaning, which makes up a complete diet – the spherical geometry (cf. P. Plichta). The structural composition of matter obeys strict mathematical laws. High order in food means high quality food. Meat has a very complex structure of the highest order, is therefore also particularly valuable (but only eaten in moderation and in high quality), but means a considerable extra effort for the organism to convert this. But every plant also has a (simpler) ordered molecular structure, which is why it should not be cooked heavy and too long. The loss of ingredients (vitamins) plays a rather subordinate role compared to the loss of structure. However, this should not lead to the conclusion that raw food is the better choice. These structures are almost impossible to break down by the organism, but only by the physiological intestinal flora, which is why the proportion of raw food should not be too high.

Food as an organising element in the treatment therefore has a double meaning.

Information

Popp et al. were able to prove the high content of biophotons in biodynamic vegetables compared to other varieties. Photons act as information carriers.

They are able to trigger 1 chemical reaction in 1 nanosecond. This are 1 billion reactions in 1 second. This extremely high speed is necessary to control the 30,000-100,000 chemical reactions per second (!) in each body cell. With the intake of food we take over stored life information of the sunlight, which changes our metabolism depending on the composition of the food. In this context, oil seeds are of particular importance because they provide us with the unsaturated fats and at the same time contain electrons that have the specific solar spin. Thus they enable us to absorb the necessary life information of the sunlight and to induce increased potential vortices.

Depending on the composition of the food, the metabolism is switched to anabolic or catabolic. The regulator in healthy people is the food itself. One can therefore formulate:

Food is a strong metabolic regulator and has a hormone-like (controlling) effect.

The mass fraction in matter is extremely small anyway. It is only 0.00000001%! The "rest" of 99.9999999% is energy and information (interaction quants). Every vitamin, every mineral is in reality only an information carrier. Theoretically, it would therefore be sufficient if we only took 1 molecule of a vitamin. However, we know from experience that we need a certain minimum amount every day. This is due to the high ***coherence*** that is necessary for the transmission of information. This is increased by the number of identical molecules. Furthermore, the relationship

$$\text{Amount of information (bit)} \approx \frac{1}{\text{degree of order}}$$

This shows that a high degree of order is necessary for good information transmission. The primary concern of every therapist should therefore be to raise the degree of order (which is the real concern of a diet). Only then can the organism be enabled to carry out its regulatory processes without errors again.

By applying the 3rd law of thermodynamics, living systems achieve this goal without effort, by reducing excitation and "returning to the quantum-mechanical ground state" acc. B. Pointer. This increases the degree of order all by itself.

Diseases that show a high degree of loss of order (e.g. cancer) only require megadoses of stabilising vitamins and minerals because information can still be transferred via the associated improvement in coherence and thus influence the metabolism. If, however, the degree of order were primarily increased, this could be done without. The supply of medicines that is actually necessary would be considerably reduced.

Holistic reflections

We live in a polar world. Complete descriptions of reality are only possible if the two polar extremes are sought out and placed in relation to each other. "Warm" can only be understood if it is placed in relation to "cold". It is the same with nutrition. Today's dietary guidelines, such as those published by the DGE (German Society for Nutrition), are based on ingredients and quantities. This is the western materialistic view of the world. Eastern ideas have always been based on the idea of life energy, qi, or in more modern terms, *bioplasm* (information). Through global communication, both notions now merge to form the necessary polarity between mass and energy. Apparently we have been following a "minority" for too long and have overlooked the majority.

The two polar extremes together form matter, which basically consists of the trinity of *mass, energy and information*. Mass and energy are therefore the extremes of one polarity. They are therefore the same. The structure that emerges from both is determined solely by information. The tissue structure of our organism is therefore also determined entirely by the information contained in the genetic material. Mass and energy only play the role of extras. This requires a constant flow of information, which comes from the *outside* from the sun photons and is stored in the potential vortices, and is effected *inside* via laser-like photon radiation from the DNA. Photons trigger the metabolic functions.

For us, the intake of food represents a supply of foreign information that the organism has to deal with, just as with any other foreign stimulus.

Every piece of information embodies a partial aspect of creation. The more natural its origin, the more harmonious its effects. With the intake of food, we create a "sounding board" within ourselves, through which a cosmic active principle, a partial aspect of the idea of creation and thus of the blueprint can be realised (via oscillation coupling with potential vortices). Every artificial destruction of an original substance, e.g. in order to extract *ingredients*, leads to a disharmonious product, because it only contains partial information of the whole (compare aristolochic acid!). In the best case, a strong stimulus can be set that becomes a healing impulse. However, this requires a good *regulatory ability*. However, the opposite effect can also occur if this is greatly reduced. The intake of nutritional supplements should also be considered under this aspect.

A food can have a synergistic effect, in that it supports a certain metabolic state (e.g. anabolic in acute inflammations), or an antagonistic effect, in that it has a balancing effect. The associated supply of mass recedes numerically far into the background (the ratio is actually only 1 to 1 billion interaction quanta). In addition, only a maximum of 1/3 of the energy requirement can be covered by food anyway. At least 2/3 comes from ambient energy (neutrinos). This ratio increases to the extreme under certain stress situations. Migratory birds, for example, obtain only about one thousandth of their required energy from food; otherwise they would not be able to cross the sea.

As part of an exhibition, a fish was shown in a hermetically sealed glass vessel, swimming around happily for 6 weeks without food or oxygen. The secret lay in a particularly energy-rich water (π-water) enriched with potential vortices, which is able to store complete life information for a long time.

Other examples are people who, under supervision, did not eat food or drink water (!) for an extremely long time and yet showed hardly any signs of exhaustion (compare Therese Neumann von D-Konnersreuth). These few examples are food for thought for an attempt at a different approach to nutrition. There are currently several new approaches in science that are worth taking a closer look at.

First, there is the biophoton research of F. A. Popp, about which very remarkable things have already been reported in the past, which will not be repeated here.
Then there is the vortex research by K. Meyl, with which energy transfer processes can be better understood. Here we are dealing with longitudinal waves, which represent the hitherto missing polar component to the known transverse waves and are also called *scalar waves*. *Vortices* can be described as the archetypes of life.

Furthermore, we are becoming increasingly aware that our universe is constructed according to strict mathematical laws (cf. P. Plichta) and is always expressed in a quadruplicity, which, however, is not always the same.

Furthermore, we are becoming increasingly aware that our universe is constructed according to strict mathematical laws (cf. P. Plichta) and is always expressed in a fourfoldness, which, however, constantly interacts with the the spirit of the Creator (W. Pauli, M. Luescher).

This has far-reaching consequences for us, because in the future we should apply other systems of order that correspond to the universal laws, but are at the same time multidimensional. Such a model, which excellently meets all requirements, is the Luescher cube, into which all aspects of life can be exactly inserted. This allows us to judge whether certain statements are correct or incomplete.

For nutritional theory, therefore, all 4 basic foods should *always* be considered *simultaneously* and thus in their *interactions.* However, only 3 are known (protein, fat, carbohydrates) because food no. 1, the water, is forgotten. But after all, water is cooked with, which changes the food and thus its effect on the organism (cf. Fig. 28 page 139).

Today we are at a crossroads. The overwhelmingly high number of chronically ill people calls for a solution. We cannot expect any new impulses from the hitherto customary, materialistic view of science. This is not least due to the still valid dualism, the "either-or", which can be driven to extremes by reductionist thinking. Only with fuzzy logic, through the "either-or" can opposites be overcome.

We have to decide:
  - **Do we want to continue as before and only "manage" the increasingly growing number of chronically ill people, since we have no solution to the problem?**

  - **Or are we prepared to look for new ways through fundamental rethinking?**

The concept of the human being as a *complex information-processing system* that has the ability to *organise itself through regulatory processes* and is at the same time a *spiritual being with a high degree of individuality and creativity* is clearly emerging on the horizon. From this perspective, we could in future look at the effects of our diet, with which we intervene in a controlling way in our organism.

New impulses
One of the main concerns of nutrition should be to replenish the depots of regulators, which is best achieved through a rhythm of regulation and

counter-regulation, of stress and relief. For this purpose, artificial stresses are created by the type of food, as in interval training.

In *healthy people*, other criteria must be used for *nutritional recommendations* than in chronically ill people, because healthy people adapt to different stimuli through the regulation of their metabolism and can therefore react differently to certain foods. It is always surprising that people who do not eat in a health-conscious way, drink a lot of alcohol and smoke are relatively healthy.

However, this can be explained very well with the polar metabolic regulation. A short-term, or in small quantities, *wrong diet* can indeed be seen as a stimulus and can even promote the health potential! The metabolism is "ramped up" by the counter-regulation, which increases the readiness to defend oneself. But you should not do this for too long, because the system will break down at some point. But every "sin" in between can have this positive effect, helps the psyche and builds up regulators. This speaks very much against dogmatic, one-sided diets.

The *sick person* is characterised by the blockage of a metabolic part (anabolic or catabolic). It is now a question of seeking out the deficiency behind it and remedying it. This is where every correct *dietary recommendation* should start. All foods can be examined to see whether they support the anabolic or the catabolic metabolism and whether they warm up or cool down. For this, however, it should be known which disease belongs to which division (cf. Fig. 26 page 110).

Since about 80% catabolic diseases (from cardiovascular to cancer) are prevalent nowadays, the usual effort will be to promote anabolism and therefore use mainly such foods (see p. 147). This should not be confused with black-and-white thinking, because it is actually much more complicated than that.

Characteristics of the different metabolic conditions
A chronic disease can be characterised by a predominance of the catabolic metabolic state, because there is increased catabolic activity, or a decreased anabolic one. The reverse is true on the anabolic side. Therefore, there are initially four possibilities, 2 for the anabolic side, 2 for the catabolic side:

anabolic metabolic state

either	or
anabolic activity ↑	anabolic activity normal
catabolic activity normal	catabolic activity ↓
(acute „shock phase" acc. Selye)	(chronical sickness)

catabolic metabolic state

either	or
catabolic activity ↑	catabolic activität normal
anabolic activity normal	anabolic activity ↓
(„counter shock phase" acc. Selye)	(chronic disease)

However, foods cannot be so easily divided into anabolic or catabolic, because a slightly *catabolic* food can be regulated out by the residual regulation that is still present and thus have an *anabolic* effect. So the *dose* makes the difference.

In addition, a water-rich, anabolic food has a cooling effect, but can become a warming, catabolic food through the way it is *prepared.*

We therefore distinguish between 5 criteria of effectiveness:

strongly anabolic - anabolic - **neutral** - catabolic - strongly catabolic
S A   **A**   **N**   **C**   **S C**

It has already been explained above that food should not be considered in isolation, but in its interaction with the environment, the climate, the preparation, etc. All these accompanying factors should also be considered. All these accompanying factors should also be integrated into this system, which is no problem if "heat" and "cold" are used synonymously with catabolic and anabolic for this purpose. It makes no difference whether heat is supplied from the outside or generated internally by a catabolic metabolic activity. If the environment is warm or warm food is consumed, the organism can reduce its metabolic activity. This has a stress-reducing and relaxing effect. This is desirable in catabolic diseases. Therefore, these patients should always dress warmly.

At the same time, however, it should be kept in mind that the patients are only suffering from their illness because the **anabolic** part is blocked. So the anabolic metabolism should be stimulated at the same time via the targeted *dietary recommendations*. This procedure is recommended for all catabolic diseases. However, individuality must be taken into account!

In addition – and this is only the healing-promoting, not only supporting effect – the food should be used rhythmically in the sense of Arndt-Schulz's rule to raise the regulator levels. This means that weak stimuli are given first, which can be slowly increased as the condition improves.

Nutrition scheme for healthy people

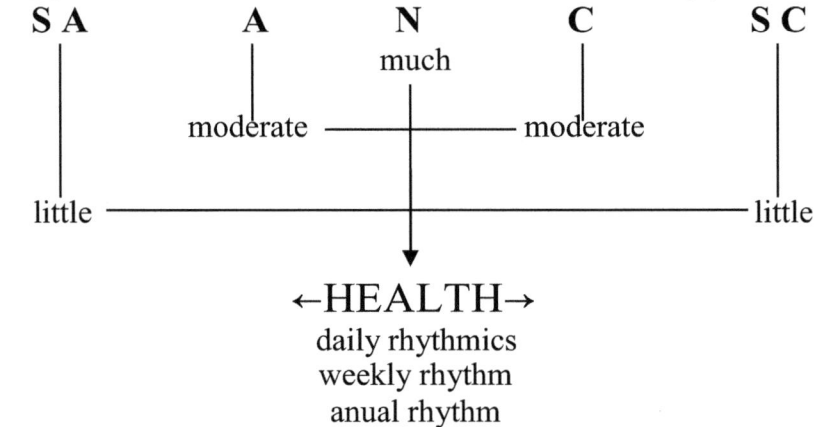

strongly anabolic - anabolic - **neutral** - catabolic - strongly catabolic

In the case of the chronically ill, specific reference is now made to the blocked metabolic part (anabolic or catabolic).
First, however, the criteria for an anabolic or catabolic state should be listed in order to be able to classify the personal, time and place-related characterristics.
The anabolic metabolism stands for regeneration and stress reduction. This should therefore always be promoted. The more the metabolic state is shifted to anabolic (protein-rich meal), the more energy is needed, which is why catabolic activity should increase (if possible at the same time).

If one leg is blocked, the other part predominates, which sometimes makes assessment somewhat difficult.

Anabolism is characterised by increased membrane permeability, which can lead to oedema. In healthy people, however, this helps to regulate the balance of juices in the tissues.

Four elemental forces of life

Of the 4 elements fire, air, earth and water, the earth (the nourishing element) and water belong to the anabolic side. The swelling of the streams to the point of flooding regulates the moistening of the earth and thus creates the basis for plant growth. However, sun (fire) is also needed for this, as well as oxygen (the counterpart of the anabolic hydrogen), which embodies the catabolic side. As long as these elementary forces can balance each other out and a constant change is possible, the conditions for growth and flourishing are optimal (cf. fig. 11 page 61). The problems only begin when the rain no longer alternates with sunshine, when flooding turns into a catastrophic flood, or when drought and dryness occur due to the incessant sunshine. The reason always lies in the loss of rhythm, the constant change.

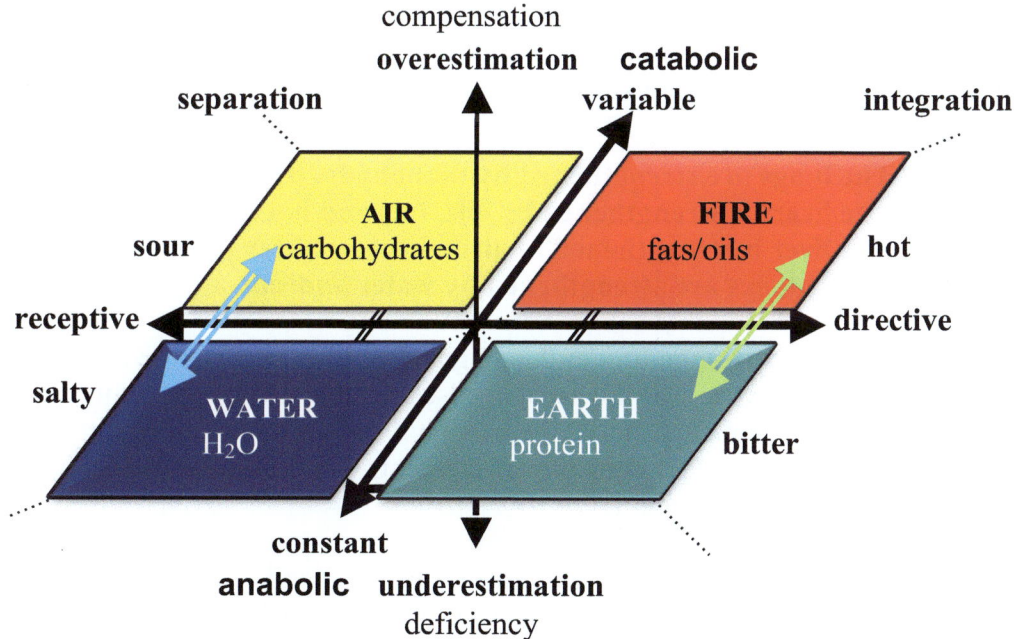

Fig. 28: Interactions of the 4 basic foods

This illustration shows very well what effects a one-sided diet can have. Life oscillates between the 4 elements and demands variety. The following interesting correlations can be seen

- carbohydrates and fats have a *catabolic* effect (each in itself).
- carbohydrates with (much) water have a *neutral* effect.
- water-rich food and protein have an *anabolic* effect.
- oil with protein has a *neutral* effect (compare Budwig)
- water and oils have an *integrating* effect (they dissolve substances)
- carbohydrates and proteins have a *separating* effect.

People who suffer from heat intolerance (too much heat) should orientate themselves on the left sagittal arrow. For them, water-containing carbohydrates (fruit, vegetables) are best suited to cool down (also teas!).

The right sagittal arrow should be followed by those who suffer from heat deficiency and freeze easily. The Budwig oil-protein diet has a neutral effect on metabolism. The more fats are supplied (in combination with protein), the more energy is released. If this energy is not used, storage fats are synthesised, which leads to weight gain.

As is well known, organs can also be assigned to the four elements, which makes an extended dietary recommendation possible:

- The lungs are strengthened by carbohydr. (rice!) and acidic foods.
- The heart is strengthened by oils, fats and hot spices.
- The liver is strengthened by proteins and bitter foods.
- The kidneys are strengthened by water and salt.

But polarity (corresponding to the diagonal) is also important when it comes to avoiding stress. Cardiovascular diseases are associated with the fire element. Heart patients should therefore not take in too much water.
Lung patients correspond to the air element, which is why they should not consume too much protein.

Liver patients belong to the earth element and should rather avoid carbohydrates because of the danger of fatty liver (NAFLD).
In this classification, too, the polar partner is usually responsible for the lack of balance (deficiency), which is why the deficiencies should be looked at first.

Schedule A:

Decreased anabolic activity is characterised by the features of catabolism (a lot of heat, lack of coolness and increased dampness):

- **restlessness, nervousness**
- **night sweats**
- **hot soles of the feet (at night)**
- **sleep disturbances**
- **internal heat**
- **thirst, dry mouth**
- **jumpiness**
- **fast, hasty speech**
- **susceptibility to stress**
- **tendency to anger**
- **little reserves**
- **dizziness**
- **headaches**
- **weight problems ($\uparrow$ or $\downarrow$)**

Schedule B:

Decreased catabolic activity is characterised by the features of anabolism (lots of dampness and coolness, lack of heat):

- **fatigue**
- **feeling of heaviness**
- **susceptibility to infections**
- **lack of concentration**
- **listlessness, slow movement and speech**
- **anxiety, resignation**
- **feeling of fullness, flatulence**
- **cravings for sweets and stimulants**
- **change in stool consistency**
- **no recovery through sleep**
- **frequent freezing, cold limbs**
- **water retention**
- **back pain that improves with exercise**
- **aversion to cold food or drink**
- **frigidity or impotence**
- **menstrual irregularities**

From this, the targeted procedure is derived in order to act on the blockage in the sense of a swing therapy and to gradually improve the self-regulation of the metabolism with the remaining residual regulation. This must be done very carefully, strictly in the sense of the Arndt-Schulz rule.

Patients with the characteristics listed in scheme A should be given primarily water-containing, cooling food in order to reduce the excessive heat. This refers to the composition of the food itself, but also to the way it is prepared. Strong heating and long cooking are then not indicated. At the same time, carbohydrates should be significantly reduced, as they prevent the release of the anabolic growth hormone. Permanent stress must also be reduced.

The *dietary recommendation* for a chronically ill person with blocked anabolic metabolism (i.e. predominance of catabolism) would therefore look like this:

Nutritional regimen for catabolic diseases

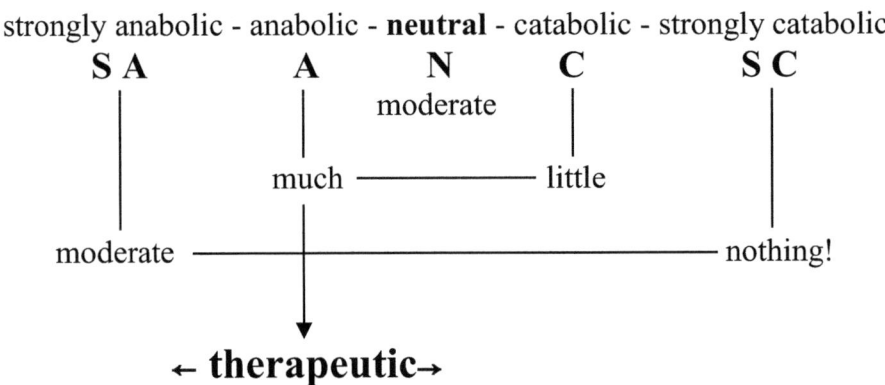

strongly anabolic - anabolic - **neutral** - catabolic - strongly catabolic

S A   **A**   **N**   **C**   **S C**

moderate

much ———— little

moderate ———————————— nothing!

← **therapeutic** →
dietary recommendation
3 days long
hot spring and summer days
high stress levels
catabolic diseases

This approach not only helps with catabolic cardiovascular diseases, chronic inflammations and even cancer, but is also suitable for hot spring and summer days. For this purpose, one orients oneself – starting from an anabolically emphasised diet – alternately to both sides, whereby the catabolic side should only be lightly touched (few carbohydrates!), depending on the severity of the illness or the environmental conditions (the colder, the more internal heat is allowed).

Another factor that must always be taken into account is the patient's level of physical exertion. Since carbohydrates are metabolised first during physical activity, the blood sugar level drops, which is why more carbohydrates can be consumed than during predominantly sedentary activity. It is also important to distinguish whether the carbohydrates are whole-grain products, which are broken down slowly, or products similar to sugar (processed flours, potatoes, cooked carrots, white sugar, peeled rice), which lead to a rapid rise in blood sugar with subsequent insulin release. This would further increase catabolism or block anabolism, which cannot be desirable.

In the approx. 20% of anabolic diseases, from asthma to rheumatism to sarcoidosis, where energy is lacking, the opposite is true. This procedure is recommended for healthy people on cold autumn and winter days. The aim here is to generate heat.

Nutritional regimen for anabolic diseases

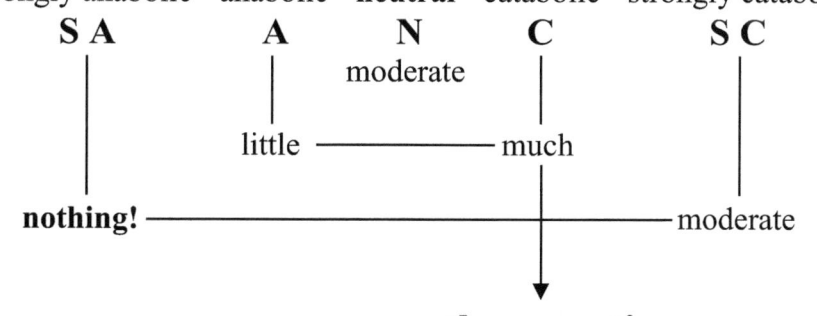

strongly anabolic - anabolic - **neutral** - catabolic - strongly catabolic

S A   **A**   **N**   **C**   **S C**

moderate

little ————————— much

nothing! —————————————— moderate

← therapeutic→
dietary recommendation
3 days
cold autumn and winter days
lack of energy
anabolic diseases

Food selection

The decisive quality feature is not primarily the ingredients, but the content of stored sun photons in the electron tori. In order to keep this as high as possible, controlled organic cultivation is to be preferred in any case and any dubious origin is to be avoided. Besides a lack of biophotons, but also herbicides and pesticides that have a destructive effect on the highly sensitive lipoproteid structures in the membranes, which is difficult to repair. In this day and age, therefore, more strict standards must be applied by the consumer. The more consistently this is done, the more likely producers will change.

In all food products, a watchful eye should be kept on the preservatives used. Preserving means adding substances that prevent oxidation. If we use these, internal cellular respiration is blocked, which in the worst case means asphyxiation of the cells, or if it does not come to that, at least energy depletion.

It is therefore important to

- **avoid anything that blocks**
- **compensate for deficiencies**
- **permanently normalise the pathological metabolic situation**
  (with loss of adaptation).

In the majority of catabolic diseases, where the anabolic limb is blocked, HGH-inhibiting carbohydrates should be avoided and anabolic foods should be consumed instead (see below).

Anabolic metabolism *inhibiting* foods

Carbohydrates, which lead to a rapid rise in blood sugar, have the greatest effect as anabolic-inhibiting foods. The associated rise in insulin levels leads to an inhibition of the anabolic metabolic regulator, the growth hormone HGH. The values can be determined via the "glycaemic index" (scale from 0 - 100). It is highest (in descending order) for

- **potatoes** (especially fried potatoes)
- **boiled carrots** (this effect does not occur raw)
- **white sugar**
- **extract flour products** (bread, pasta)
- **corn**
- **rice** (peeled)

It therefore plays an important role whether the sugar contained is released quickly or delayed (extract flour versus wholemeal products).

Foods that *promote* anabolism
include all those that have a highly complex structure (increases the degree of order). They usually require a large amount of (catabolic) energy to break them down. This is particularly the case with meat. It is the strongest anabolic food of all (compare heavy athletes).

Furthermore, all fats have an anabolic effect, saturated ones more than unsaturated ones, but only in combination with proteins (e.g. fatty meat). If fat is consumed alone, it is immediately metabolised and then has a ***catabolic*** effect.

Lipoproteins (oil-protein compounds) have a neutral effect. They can therefore be used without problems in both metabolic states and at the same time create the basis for energy absorption from sunlight.

Indirectly anabolic (via the cooling effect) are all water-rich products, such as tomatoes, cucumbers, melon, apples, etc. However, the preparation must always be taken into account. (If, for example, a baked apple is eaten, it has a catabolic effect.) These vegetables and fruits are also among the

catabolic *inhibitors.*
Other catabolic inhibiting foods include citrus fruits and bananas, yoghurt, most teas (except black tea) and mineral water.

Catabolic-*promoting* foods
include all stimulating things such as hot spices, coffee, black tea, red wine, sugar in any form, and other rapidly digestible carbohydrates such as potatoes, cooked carrots, all extract flours, husked rice and maize. Other foods can have a catabolic effect if prepared with heat. In general, therefore, it can be said:

Heat-producing foods have a catabolic effect; cold-producing foods have an anabolic effect.

This list should first clarify the principle of how to assess the effect of individual foods. Further classifications can be found in the following table or in the list according to the glycaemic index (from page 151).

Very many foods have a neutral effect and can therefore be used in both cases without any problems. These include whole foods, which can be used to create a stable basis. According to Chinese nutritional teachings, the centre is first strengthened (spleen-pancreas) in order to create a stable basis. From there, the energy is distributed further in the organism according to the rules of the 5 phases of changing.

If "the oven" is not preheated, the food cannot be broken down properly, which can lead not only to digestive disorders, but also to deficiencies and even weight gain (because of the low heat of combustion).

Assignment of food – metabolic effects

The following tables are based on the Chinese elemental diet according to B. Temelie. The allocation to organ systems can be taken from the original table of the book (see literature appendix). It should be noted that the *type of preparation* is essential, which is why the table can only give a rough overview. The more heat is added, the longer something cooks, the more catabolic it is in terms of energy input.

Besides the amount of heat added during preparation (which has a catabolic effect), another important point is the *inhibition* of metabolic regulation by certain foods. For example, all extract flours prevent a rise in anabolic activity, which has an unfavourable effect on regeneration as well as the performance of the immune system.

For reasons of space, these tables do not distinguish between catabolically active and anabolically inhibiting. Both appear in the same column.

The choice for a patient depends on the underlying disease, but above all on his heat-energy balance. The more sensitive a patient is to cold, the more catabolic foods he needs, but of these, all anabolic-inhibiting substances that drive up blood sugar should be avoided!

It should be noted, however, that a disease of the thyroid gland can make the allocation difficult. A blatant iodine deficiency, which by the way is not only found in the mountains, automatically leads to hypothyroidism, which cannot be counteracted with catabolic-enhancing foods alone. Here, a targeted substitution with natural iodine from algae (e.g. brown algae kelp) is absolutely necessary. The dose depends on the heart rate and the inner well-being, which should set in after a short time. If restlessness and nervousness occur, it must be reduced.

Effect of food on the metabolism

strongly anabolic	anabolic	neutral	catabolic	strongly catabolic
G r a i n (integral)				
wheat bran	wheat buckwheat barley	bulgur couscous spelt amaranth cuinoa rye millet wholemeal rice	green spelt sweet rice oats	**all** **extract.** **flours** **in pasta** **and bred** **corn** **white** **rice**
F r u i t s				
pineapple **kiwi** **rhubarb** **lemon** **honeydew melon** **persimmon** **mango** **papaya** **watermelon**	apple cranberry strawberry blueberry blackcurrant sour cherry tangerine orange clementine gooseberry grapefruit quince banana pear	blackberry raspberry date fig plum	pomegranate kumquat plum apricot sweet cherry corinth peach sultana	**dry fruits**
V e g e t a b l e s				
	chickpea sweet pepper black salsify celery asparagus spinach courgettes cress white radish	lentils		

Effect of food on the metabolism

strongly anabolic	anabolic	neutral	catabolic	strongly catabolic
Vegetables				
mung beans-	alfa alfa-	nettle	brussels spr.	**cooked**
sprout	sprout	iceberg lett.	fennel	**carots**
sorrel	legume	endive	onion	**potatoe**
tomato	sprouts	lamb's lett.	leek	
cucumber	nasturtium	beetroot	horseradish	
	sour cabbage	green bean		
	bean sprouts	peas		
	artichoke	pumpkin		
	chicory	carrot raw		
	lettuce	kohlrabi		
	dandelion	red cabb.		
	radicchio	w. cabbage		
	rocket	savoycabb.		
	aubergine	yam		
	cauliflower	radish black		
	(broccoli)	beans		
	chinese cabb.	peas		
Fish				
caviar	oysters	perch	eel	
crab	squid	trout	prawns	
seaweed		halibut	lobster	
crayfish		carp	crawfish	
mussels		salmon	cod	
			anchovy	
			plaice	
			tuna	
			smoked fish	
Meat				
	duck	chicken	all grilled	
	goose		meat sorts	
	turkey		all game	
	quail		lamb	
	rabbit		goat	
	beef		salami, ham	

Effect of food on the metabolism

strongly anabolic	anabolic	neutral	catabolic	strongly catabolic
Milk products				
yoghurt	soured milk cream cheese curd kefir sour cream whipped cream	butter cow's milk	sheep cheese goat's cheese goat's milk Harz cheese Muenster cheese Parmesan cheese	**blue cheese**
Beverages				
Mineral water **cold water** **Prosecco**	bread drink Champagne Prosecco white wine wheat beer Altbier/Pils corn tea mauve tea melissa tea green tea orange blossom tea peppermint tea apple/pear juice hot water	rosehip tea liquorice tea grape juice	black tea cherry juice coffeinfree coffee red wine Port wine liqueur honey wine rice wine fennel tea	**high per-** **centage** **alcohol** **Yogi tea**
Other				
salt **soy sauce** **agar agar**	sage soy tofu cashew nuts all oils olives avocado champignon	yeast saffron vanilla hazel nuts wood mushr. eggs miso molasses whole c. sug. seeds nuclears	basil savory curcuma poppy oregano rosmary thyme juniper cinnamon walnut peanuts chestnut	**chili** **cayenne** **curry** **ingwer** **garlic** **pepper** **allspice**

The following table clearly shows how the blood sugar changes. The "glycaemic index", a functional quantity, is used as an evaluation standard for the foods. This provides more clarity about the inhibitory effects on anabolic metabolism. The value should be as low as possible.

Effect of food on blood sugar

recommended:

Bread and cereal products:

Wholemeal bread	50
Bread made from shredded wheat	50
Bread made from oats and bran	50
Wholemeal muesli, no added sugar	50

Rice and noodles:

Wholemeal rice	50
Wholemeal pasta	45

Vegetables:

Green peas	45
Red and green beans	40
Dried pulses	40
Raw carrots	30
Artichokes	15
Aubergines	15
All types of cabbage	15
Broccoli	15
Green salad	15
Bell peppers	15
Mushrooms	15
Radish	15
Cucumber	15
Celery	15
Asparagus	15
Spinach	15
Tomatoes	15
Courgettes	15
Onions	15

avoid as far as possible:

Bread and cereal products:

White bread	95
Baguette	95
Pretzels	85
Corn chips	75
Popcorn	75
Crackers	75
Cornflakes	75
White flour and products	70
Millet	70
Cornmeal	70
Muesli with sugar	70
Grey bread	65
Rye bread made f. sourdough	55

Rice, pasta and potatoes:

Fried potatoes	95
Mashed potatoes	90
Quick-cooking rice	90
French fries	80
Rice cakes	80
White rice	70
Light noodles	65
Basmati rice	60
Wild rice	55

Vegetables:

Cooked carrots	85
Sweet corn	75
Turnips	75
Sweet potatoes	75

Fruit and nuts:

Mangoes	50	**Fruit:**	
Kiwis	50	Watermelons	70
Grapes	50	Pineapples	65
Pears	45	Raisins	65
Peaches	40	Dried fruit	65
Plums	40	Ripe bananas	60
Apples	40		
Oranges	40	**Sweet:**	
Grapefruits	25	Honey	75
Cherries	25	Refined sugar	75
Nuts	25	Chocolate bars	70
Fresh apricots	10	Jam	60
		Ice cream	60

Sweet:

Fruit juices without sugar	40	
Fruit spreads without sugar	40	
Fructose	20	

Intolerable

Fatty meat with skin
(duck, pork)
Cola, lemonade, fatty cheese

Also allowed

Lean meat and fish
Low-fat dairy products

In this table, the level of the glycaemic index plays a role on the one hand, and the amount of food on the other. If only very little is eaten from the right column, the effects are minimal.

However, the dynamics must also be taken into account. The predominantly sedentary person should eat as little as possible from the right column. The person who has a lot of exercise and does sport quickly reduces the elevated blood sugar again, so that a completely different assessment standard results here.

It should also always be pointed out in which combination the food is consumed and with which preparation. The anabolic effect increases when eating cold or drinking cold with food. The more heat is stored in the food, the easier it is to digest and break down the ingredients.

WEEKDAYS

	Mo	Tu	We	Th	Fr	Sa	Su
	neutral	**catabolic-effective**			**anabolic-effective**		
Nutrition	fasting	<< carbohydrates >>			<< proteins >>		
Cereals	(rice)	barley	millet	rye	oats	maize	spelt
Planets	moon	Mars	Mercury	Jupiter	Venus	Saturn	(Sun)
Aspect	water	struggle	above-below	generous	growing	find meaning	light
Food	- . -	<< grilled, roasted, hot >>			<< water-contain.dishes,soups >>		
Spices	- . -	<< sour/hot >>			<< sour/salty >>		
Alcoh.drinks	- . -	<< red wine >>			<< white wine >>		
Movement	rest	<< sports >>			<< gymnastics >>		
Psyche	harmony	<< conflict resolution >>			<< structure, constructive >>		
Music	meditation	<< rock >>			<< classic >>		
Colours	green	<< red >>			<< blue >>		
Temperat.	indifferent	<< warm >>			<< cold >>		
Water	washing	<< bathing >>			<< shower >>		
Scavencher	- . -	- . -	- . -	- . —	+	+	+
Minerals	- . -	<< ca/pot./cu >>			<< sod./mg/zn >>		
Hormones	- . -	<< progesterone/T3,T4 >>			<< oestrogens >>		
Hormones	- . -	<< cortisol/T3,T4 >>			<< testosterone >>		
LSIT	MRT 503	<< perman. stress reduction >>			<< constitution support >>		
Phytoph.	- . -	-	-	-	+	+	+

Table 2: Life-Rhythm-Therapy LRT

Comment:
These recommendations apply to the relatively healthy person and serve for general strengthening and disease prophylaxis.

In *chronically ill people*, the metabolic state must first be determined (anabolic/catabolic). The further procedure depends on this:
- In *catabolic* patients, initially <u>only anabolic support</u> for 4 weeks,
- in *anabolic* patients, <u>catabolic support</u>.

Initially, therefore, orientate only on the left or right side (anabolic patients on the left, catabolic patients on the right). After that, 1 day per week is added from the other reaction layer until they can take up the normal rhythm after 7 weeks.

Aim of a dietary recommendation

The first question is what can and what should be achieved?
- **life energy increased** (assertiveness)
- **more life information absorbed** (vitality)
- **quality of life increased** (joy)
- **centring in the middle improved** (stability/resilience)
- **the regulators increased** (higher resistance)
- **regulation improved** (rapid adaptation)
- **regeneration promoted** (best aging)
- **foci of disease healed** (recovery)
- **the degree of order increased** (higher health potential)

Nutritional recommendations must not be dogma. We live in a polar world. Good times alternate with bad. Healthy food can certainly alternate with "unhealthy". This is another way to improve resistance. The ability to adapt must be trained. This increases resilience.

But not only the *type* of food, also *fullness and emptiness* should alternate. A "savings day", or even a fasting day per week, fits perfectly into the overall concept. The joy of eating, the ambience – everything should be drawn on.

The orientation of the dishes should always have the centre, the balance, in mind, around which variations are made. Cooked neutral integral dishes (e.g. rice, amaranth, millet, oats, spelt), sweetened with fruit, which strengthen the central organs pancreas (controls digestion) and spleen (controls blood and juices). Therefore, the "accompanying music" is grouped according to the external conditions. This depends on whether the anabolic or the catabolic metabolism is to be stimulated.

In today's stressful times, it is usually a question of reducing catabolic stress and increasing anabolic activity, which means regeneration, building up reserves, higher immune performance and better resilience (anabolic does not only mean weight gain!). Since we have predominantly catabolic conditions (approx. 80%), most nutritional recommendations go in the same direction.

However, the stabilisation of the base should always be kept in mind in order to contain the civilisational damage.

This is not only about the intake of the vital lipoproteins, but also about a very conscientious selection of the food itself, which is becoming more and more important for us. *Every* industrial processing automatically leads to a reduction in quality. At the same time, many of the added substances cause noticeable damage to the organism, some of which is irreversible. For this reason, it is advisable to examine the sources of food carefully and not to buy anything that does not meet the requirements. This takes a little effort, but is now just as important as the right choice of food itself. Conventional sausage and similar products fall out of the equation from the outset.

A reformed dietary teaching should be open and undogmatic. Only in this way can it adapt flexibly to new findings at any time. The impulses that the new **dietary recommendations** should contain are derived from the following points:

- **Rhythm of life** (the homeostasis of the tissue is established via rhythms, cf. H. Heine, whereby strain and relief alternate with each other, cf. table LRT page 152).

- **Geometry and order** (the higher the degree of order, the more structuring the molecular geometries have, which stand in certain numerical relationships to each other and obey the quadrality on the material level, cf. P. Plichta).

- **Information and biophotons** (foodstuffs are carriers of natural imprinting information and in this way influence the metabolism, as they can set self-organisation processes in motion, cf. F. A. Popp).

- **Hub of fat metabolism** (the importance of highly unsaturated fatty acids such as cis-linoleic acid is not only of utmost importance for membrane function and thus for regeneration pro-cesses, but must be seen as a direct pathway of energy absorption through sunlight, as these act like solar batteries, cf. J. Budwig).

- **Bipolar metabolic regulation** (anabolic & catabolic metabolic processes should be united via fuzzy logic, but the contrary effects of the same food in different doses and preparations should also be recorded, cf. J. Schole).

- **Individuality and constitution** (for each person there is only one way of eating, which is right for him here and now).

- **Bioclimatic and geographical influences** (we are embedded in our environment. We are part of the whole and cannot be isolated from it. The universe is a hologram, cf. K. Wilber).

- **Fill up deficiencies** instead of fighting surpluses (do not con-fuse the superficial symptom with the cause. The cause is hidden and only arises through a deficiency, which can show itself on different levels, cf. B. Koehler)

Practical application

The initially complicated presentation of various interactions that have to be taken into account when *recommending nutrition* turns out to be quite simple in practice after a short period of familiarisation.

First of all, the *daily workload* is considered (much or little physical exercise, stress load or not, etc.), then the *environmental conditions* (warm or cold, rain, wind, etc.) and also the *inner sensation* (heat or cold, tiredness, etc.) according to the classification "anabolic" or "catabolic".
In chronically ill patients, the *rhythm* should be included in further considerations, either anabolic or catabolic stressed.

In any case, a stable basis is created via *cooked integral cereal porridge* (not to be confused with wholemeal!), on which a metabolism-influencing diet can be built.
When using *wholemeal products*, it is important to remember that they can only be tolerated without problems if there is *no leaky gut*. If there is an increased permeability of the intestine, there may be considerable digestive problems, which are, however, a good diagnostic indicator. In this case, colostrum, activated charcoal, volcanic rock (e.g. KlinSiMag®) and krill oil, which contains a lot of lecithin, can be used successfully.

Another reason for intolerance may be phytates (derivatives of phytic acid). This is especially true for soy. These act as anti-nutrients and prevent the absorption of important minerals.
Furthermore, the plants' defence substances against predators (lectins) can cause problems. A particular representative is WGA (wheat germ agglutinin), which can lead to antibody formation and thus cause severe wheat intolerance. The aggressive lectins are normally rejected by an intact intestinal mucosa and thus do not burden the organism.

But it is not only leaky gut that can lead to intruding. If the mucus pathway is not intact because Akkermansia muciniphilia bacteria are missing or the lamina propria has defects, the natural barrier is also partially removed. Glucosamine (e.g. Glucosa-K2®) has proven effective here.

If the blood group is sensibly included in the considerations, then with BG A the emphasis is on grains and vegetables, with BG 0 on protein.

If there is an energy deficiency and/or the daily workload is very energy-consuming, then the foods (or their preparation) are selected according to whether they are catabolically effective. In the other case of increased catabolic activity, the opposite is true (much more common). The goal of the dietary recommendation (according to the above list) should be kept firmly in mind: Comprehensive well-being and enjoyment of life have top priority.

Since we find degenerative diseases in most cases today, or should protect ourselves from them, it is advisable to observe the 10 points of prevention or treatment of civilisation diseases in any case, in order to reactivate the "sun collectors" in us (see page 37).

Since the nutritional basis is the *oil-protein diet*, some important details should be discussed here, as they were worked out by Johanna Budwig.
All preparations of lipoproteins should be made fresh before each meal. Otherwise, due to rapid oxidation, the products may not only be worthless, but may even have harmful effects on the liver.

The *proteins* used are primarily those that contain sulphur-containing amino acids. These are curd cheese and other types of cheese, leek vegetables, leeks, chives, onions and garlic.

Oils containing polyunsaturated fatty acids, especially linoleic acid, are used as fats. It is contained in linseed oil, but also in krill oil, sunflower oil, soybean oil, maize oil, poppy seed oil, walnut oil, but not in peanut oil! Linseed oil and krill oil also contain linolenic acid, which is very important for the brain and nerves. Freshly (!) ground linseed or linomel (linseed coated with honey) is highly recommended, especially for women (oestrogen effect).

Carbohydrates should be given mainly as natural complex sugars, as found in sweet fruits, dates, figs, pears, apples, grapes, berries, etc. But be careful: since fructose does not require insulin to be absorbed into the cells, increased consumption can lead to non-alcoholic fatty liver disease (NAFLD), which is difficult to diagnose. Sweet fruit should therefore only be consumed in moderation, or with sufficient physical exercise!

Beta-carotene in raw (!) carrots, as well as B vitamins in buttermilk and whey, and good (live) yeast have a supporting effect.

In any case, lactic fermented vegetable juices should be drunk at the same time (1 bottle daily) to better eliminate the precipitated fat deposits.

The lipoproteids are prepared by mixing 3 large tbsp. fresh (!) linseed oil with at least 3 tbsp. goat's or sheep's milk to form an emulsion (wooden spoon, no machines!) and adding 125 g organic low-fat quark. Then 2 table-spoons of linomel (females only) can be added as well as walnuts and 1 tea-spoon of good honey.
Herbs, spices and onions can also be added to the lipoproteid cream and the whole thing can be individually refined to make it tastier.

The oil-protein diet replaces a meal and can be taken every morning, in severe cases also several times a day. In the case of bile disorders, it may be necessary to take ursodeoxycholic acid in the form of Ursofalk 500, as this important bile acid is essential for resorption. Further suggestions can be taken from the book "Oil-Protein Diet" by J. Budwig.
It should be noted, however, that not all patients can tolerate this diet. If viral diseases have occurred in the past that were toxic to the liver, e.g. hepatitis A, B, C or Eppstein-Barr, certain enzyme systems that are neces-sary for processing may be blocked. If this is the case, there will be rancid secretions through the skin as a sign of intolerance, and it must be avoided.

General recommendations

- The "how" of food intake plays just as big a role as the "what". Besides an ambience that appeals to the senses, the inner attitude towards food plays a major role.

- Eat at least 1 warm meal a day (this can also be soups). Meal times at fixed times if possible, so that the body can adjust, not too heavy in the evening (no protein, but also no salads that can ferment!) and eating too late (not after 6.00 p.m.).

- The more severely ill a patient is, the smaller the portions should be, but eat more frequently (possibly up to 30 times a day) small bites until there is an improvement).

- Every food should be as natural as possible (according to Kollath) and prepared gently. This applies not only to vegetables, but also for oils, which should not be heated. Microwave ovens and motor-driven kitchen appliances (electron robbers!) should be avoided.

- The proportion of fresh vegetable food (salad, fruit, vegetables) should be as high as possible (approx. 2/3), but must be adapted to the more or less intact digestive function and should then be mainly steamed or gently cooked. In winter, the proportion of raw vegetables must be significantly lower than in summer because of the cooling effect.

- Pork sausages with added nitrate or curing salt containing nitrate should be strictly avoided, as should pork itself.

- The intestinal flora can be supported by acidic dextrorotatory milk products (in small quantities, otherwise they have a slyming effect).
  All lactic acid fermented products (e.g. whey, buttermilk, but also vegetable juices) are recommended, as well as "Kanne bread drink". Milk should be avoided (also by children), as it is the most common allergen. It contains growth factors for calves that put stress on the immune system.

- Ensure a sufficient intake of omega-3 fatty acids, but if possible in combination with protein as an oil-protein diet according to Budwig (see there). Alternatively, krill oil, which also has high lecithin content, is recommended.

- Animal or hardened fats and heated oils (frying, deep fryer) should be avoided as far as possible. Coconut fat can be used for frying or butter. The total amount of fat (not heated) should not exceed 60-80 g/day and should be consumed with only a few carbohydrates.

- The constant supply of silica (not calcium!) is essential for the function of the basic system (according to Pischinger) and bone formation. Silica is found in larger quantities in millet, oats and barley.

- When taking in minerals, attention should be paid to their metabolic effects (cf. sub-chapter "Electrolytes"). Due to the calcium surplus that is usually present, magnesium should be given special attention.

- The daily amount of fluid should only be covered by purified water (e.g. with a carbon block filter) and should be determined individually.

Drink mineral water only on hot days, do not drink juices too often, avoid soft drinks completely. Alcohol consumption should be limited, as it puts a strain on the liver's vital detoxification function, among other things.

- Zinc is eminently important for the immune system, but is only found in sufficient quantities in meat and oysters.

Nutrition and cancer

First of all, the guidelines of the "General Recommendations" should be followed. In addition:

- Carbohydrates should be drastically reduced so that the insulin level remains low; otherwise the defence function is slowed down (by inhibiting HGH). According to W. Zabel, fasting blood sugar should not exceed 80-90 mg%. Carbohydrates that should be significantly reduced for at least 6 weeks include sugar, cooked carrots, potatoes, all white flour products (bread, pasta, etc.), rice and maize.

- The oil-protein diet described above as part of the 10-point programme for civilisation diseases has top priority and is an indispensable part of every cancer diet! In severe cases, it can be taken up to 3 times a day.

- Wheat bran has proven to be very helpful and also leads to improved intestinal cleansing.

- Meat is indispensable for the organism because of its high degree of order, especially for blood group 0. However, it should only be eaten in the very best organic quality and, because of the putrefactive products (ammoniac!) and the resulting toxic liver load, not too often and only in combination with salad, vegetables and acidic dairy products; pork should not be eaten under any circumstances.

- When taking minerals, attention should be paid to their anabolic effect (Mg, Na, Zn) and should prefered in opposite to those with a catabolic effect (Ca, K, Cu). Therefore, the intake of magnesium is advisable, but calcium should be avoided at all costs (which is found in large quantities in broccoli, for example)!

- Cortisone or thyroid hormones have a catabolic effect and should be avoided if possible (except in the case of insufficiency of the endocrine glands, or lymphomas and sarcomas, as these are ana-bolic).

- Water intake can be supported by water with healing properties. So-called π-water has proved its worth, but also other oxygen-enriched preparations (Futomat). Among the natural waters, Dunaris sparkling water and Haderheck water deserve special mention. Only drink freshly hand-squeezed juices (vegetable juices). As teas are favourable corn tea (not too often), green tea, red bush tea, Hapargophytum tea.

- Green leafy vegetables, raw (!) carrots, citrus fruits in particular, tomatoes, cabbage, apples, raw sauerkraut, kohlrabi, cress, white radish, asparagus, wheat bran, figs, peach pits as well as almonds (chew 1 of them every hour) have a particularly favourable effect on inhibiting cancer growth.

- Some types of mushrooms (including shiitake) also have a very beneficial effect.

  - Red Korean ginseng in sufficiently high doses has a strong anabolic and tonic effect.

- Smoking must be stopped and staying in smoky rooms must be avoided.

- Ensure warm clothing and warm surroundings so that the organism reduces its catabolic (heat-producing) activity.

- Food should be used rhythmically as a stimulus. For this purpose, after the 6-week conversion phase, light loads of integral carbo-hydrates are introduced in a weekly rhythm.

Further advice can be taken from the book by the author "Cancer – a cureable disease" (see references).

Conclusions on nutrition

Nutrition could actually become a highly effective component of any treatment or health maintenance if there is a thorough rethink here. For this to happen, however, the purely material view would have to be expanded to include the concept of quality. The "how" of food intake can be stronger, positive information than the food itself, if it is done with an altered, positive consciousness.

Without a correct dose-effect relation and in the absence of a polarity relation, no exact scientific statement about food intake is possible.

The often opposing effects of food can only be understood through certain interactions. To grasp these in their entirety becomes possible through the three-component theory of metabolic regulation according to J. Schole. It is therefore worthwhile to increasingly integrate this field into medicine.

7. Fundamentals of Life-supporting Medicine

It sounds presumptuous to want to present the basics of medicine in a handbook intended for practical use, and to do so with a great many new facts and aspects. This could not succeed even if the approach were analytical. Here, the opposite approach will be taken: First the general overview with a unified concept, then some necessary details. The reader can then decide for himself which accompanying literature he would like to read in greater depth.

What did not exist in medicine before was the red guide that would enable the student as well as the doctor to have targeted and immediate access to data needed in the particular case of their patients. Data that allow an assessment of which influences (lifestyle, diet, certain treatments, etc.) have had a *life-supporting* effect, or an *inhibiting* effect on the life process. Due to this omission, many difficulties arise today in the assessment of disease patterns, but also in finding the appropriate therapy.

It would be much easier if we were primarily concerned with the principles of life and the various influences on them, instead of with the complexity of the organism, which can never be grasped.

We could focus on the inner and outer factors with which our body interacts. Then we can keep track of everything. Let's just admit that the immune system has stored programmes for *all* external attacks with which it can react effectively. So let's not constantly interfere with our "anti's" to stop some natural process that we don't understand anyway. Let us rather deal with the influences on the regulatory mechanisms.

We should be very careful about any separation and division of the organism into individual components, because it is always an artificial one. It forms a unity. Similarly, it is impossible to separate mind-soul-body. It is better to think in terms of functional units and systems, but on several levels.

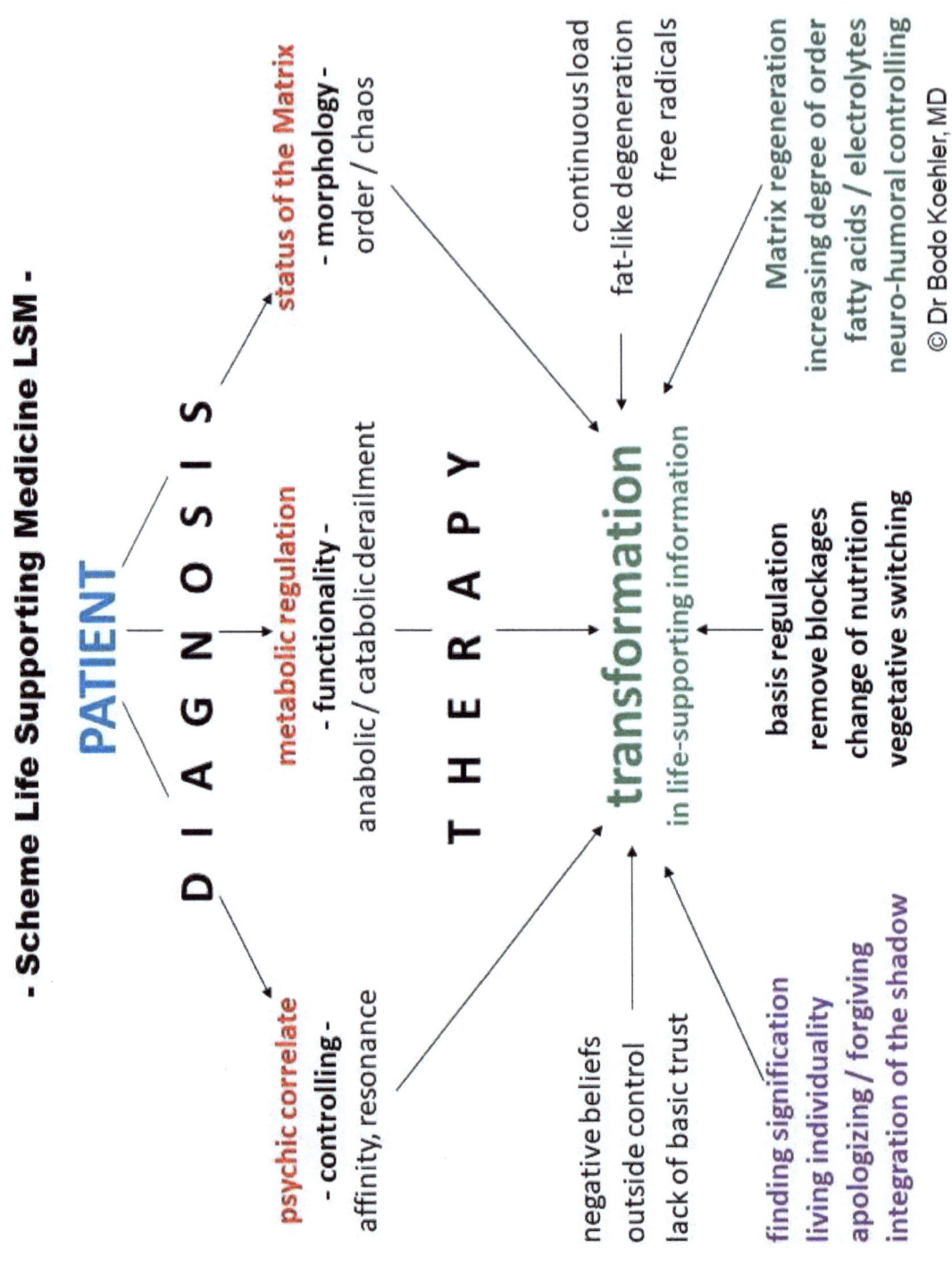

Fig. 29: Scheme of life-supporting medicine

For this reason, we should first look at 3 areas in each patient:
- **psychological correlate of the disease**
- **metabolic state and its derailment**
- **condition of the matrix and organ cells**

We can also call these 3 criteria ***control, functionality and morphe*** (cf. Fig. 29).

It is also time that the importance that matter has had up to now is shifted. If until now mass has been favoured, this is put into perspective when one considers that it makes up just 0.00000001% of our material reality. However, in order to create something in reality, ***information*** is necessary (the ***idea***). But this can only have an effect (bring something into form) if there is resonance with similar patterns. Every disease originated because of certain information, because there was an affinity. Only if we deal more intensively with all 3 areas, we work on the cause.

Derived from holistic scientific findings, we come to the following statements relevant to medicine:

*1. Our Creator in his trinity creates matter in its quaternity. The **idea** remains permanently connected to it as information. Through our attention (sharpness) we make a selection from innumerable possibilities (fuzziness) and thus fix our reality. A change of this (focus of disease) can only take place through a transformation of the triggering information.*

*2. The (extended) concept of matter includes **mass, energy and information** (spirit). Matter can be understood as a particle as well as a wave (field). The **structure** is subject to the **law of four**, a strictly geometrical construction plan according to mathematical-musical laws and can be regarded as a **sound body.***

*3. Our reality can only be properly grasped in its **polarity.** Life means **asymmetry,** which makes it possible **to gain experience.** Illness arises from a dysbalance of the two polar pols to the point of disharmony, which reveals a **deficiency.** Behind this is often the rejection of certain aspects of life ("shadows"), due to unresolved conflicts.*

*4. Spirit – soul – body with all their interactions form a unity. The human being can be understood as a **complex information-processing, self-regulating system inspired by the spirit.** Healing is seen as an **active process of consciousness** of the patient and implies the intention to reintegrate into the cosmic order and to dissolve wrong behavioural patterns.*

*5. The performance of the body's cells is tied to the **functioning of the basic regulatory system** (the matrix) in which they are embedded. Here the information levels are linked via **complex networked control circuits**. The quality of the information transmission depends on the **degree of order in the tissue** (sounding board, tones and sounds).*

*6. The **meridian system** acts as a **light conductor for the life energy Qi (bioplasm)**. The nervous system as a neuronal network is the carrier of **holographic information**. It communicates via direct current, maser impulses and scalar waves. All body zones interact with the corresponding brain areas (2nd localisation of interference fields).*

*7. The energy supply is only partially provided by food, but for the most part by direct absorption of **solar photons** as a special form of neutrinos, which are **stored by electrons** and contain necessary life information **(bioplasm).** The prerequisites for this are created via **auto-oxidation** of the omega 3 fats and sulphur-protein compounds.*

*8. Functionality is made possible by the bipolar metabolic activity (anabolic + catabolic), which must be regarded as the hub of all bodily functions. Every functional disorder is an expression of a **local cell metabolism blockade.** The primary search should always be for a **deficiency.***

*9. The material conditions for life and thus health are supported by an electrodynamic process **(electron-donor-acceptor reaction)** – brought about by potential vortices – through which metabolic regulation is made possible.*

*10. Every serious illness should always be diagnosed and treated on **all 3 levels** (psyche – cell metabolism – matrix). Only then is real healing possible. First of all, the energy balance must be normalised, whereby, in addition to the supply of highly unsaturated fats, the degradation of degenerated, solidified fats has top priority.*

Implementation in practice

Medicine must become simple and straightforward again! If you stick to the few (!) basic principles of life that our organism obeys in everyday practice, you can achieve a high level of efficiency. The most important thing is to know these and to classify malfunctions correctly. The human body works according to the same laws as life itself, because it is the expression of an active spirit. It is life. If we take the spiritual laws as a basis, then we will understand the development of diseases much better and new therapeutic approaches will open up, which are also much more cost-effective due to their effectiveness.

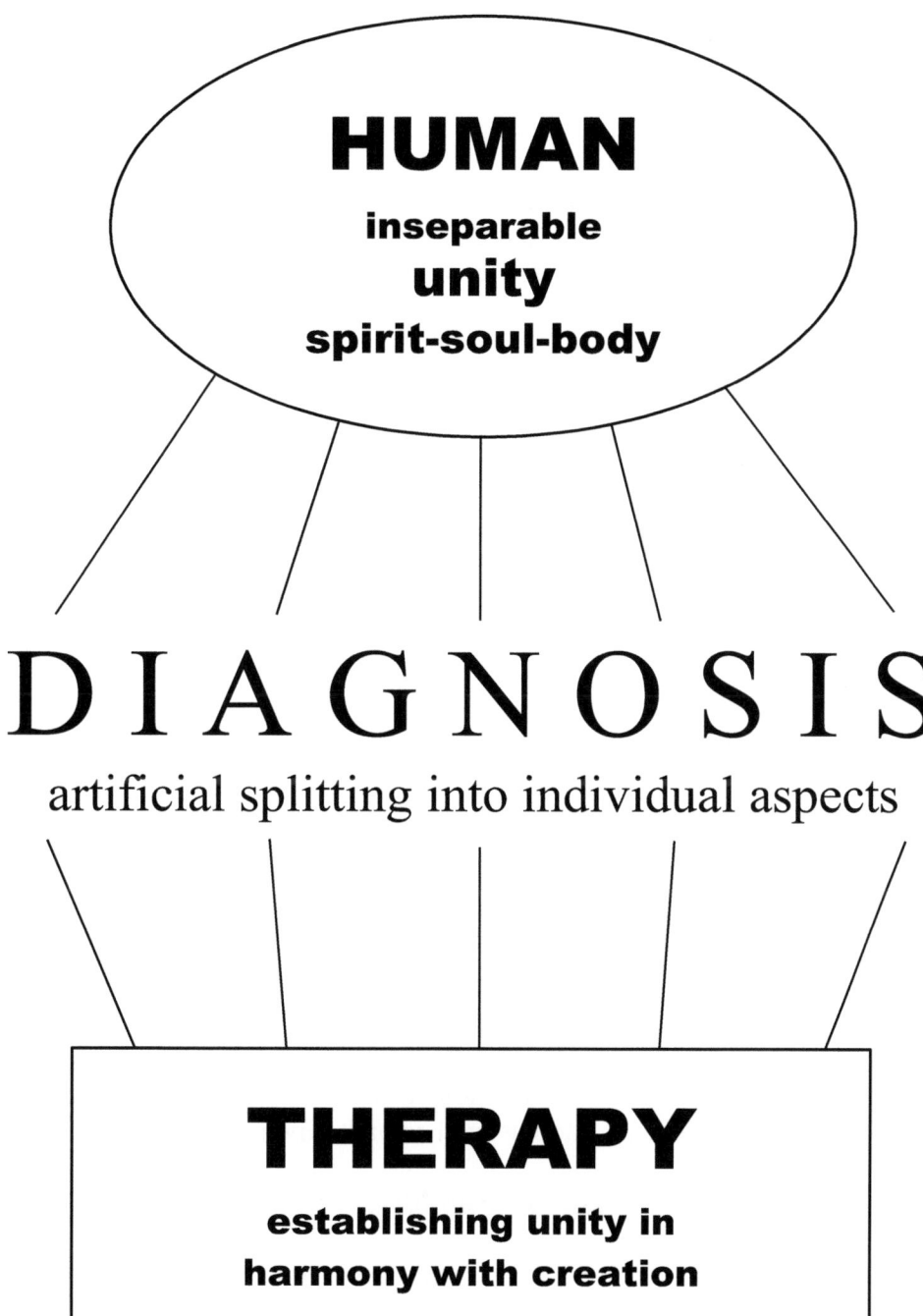

Fig. 30: The human being as an inseparable unit

Syntactics – the idea of unity

First of all, we should recognise that our entire universe is an inseparable unity. Any division into separate parts is an artificial one and can be seen as purely intellectual. Most misunderstandings of our time are based on separation and fragmentation. This must become *unification and commonality* again!

Let us try for once to preferentially see what unites us, in all areas. Just as all human beings form a whole humanity, the spirit that moves us is also a unity that connects us all. On this level, no separation is possible.

In order to get to the origin of every change (which is always a spiritual one), it would therefore make much more sense to emphasise what connects and to refrain from what separates.

Whether we are talking about our patients, whom we regard as an inseparable unity of mind-soul-body, or personal destinies, which must not be detached from our own misbehaviour – only the *unifying aspect* always leads to the holistic view we desire. The objective can be achieved through *syntactical thinking*. For this, it is necessary to complete the existing world view and thus also the human image.

Basic prerequisites for the new view are

unity of spirit-soul-body
global interconnectedness
hierarchical structures

Law of resonance

Each of our actions, each of our words, and already each of our thoughts sets an *impulse* that spreads throughout the entire universe until it encounters resonance. Then there is a reaction, which has an effect on ourselves. This is a law to which we are all subject. In this way, we create each of our life situations ourselves – good as well as bad – including illnesses!

Illness is the result of a resonance problem.

Illness therefore does not arise because we have (accidentally) become infected somewhere. The interplay of *Actio and Reactio*, in which we ourselves are actively involved, can cause it. Every impuls provokes a counter impuls.

We can become ill when we

- **disregard spiritual laws and leave the path of virtue**
- **repeatedly violate the cosmic order**
- **ignore the purpose and goal of our life**
- **live against our constitution** (asymmetry)
- **rejecting parts of life through values and judgements**
- **not filling up an existing deficit** (deficiency)
- **not controlling the input and output of our open system**
- **disregarding natural rhythms as a principle of order** (stagnation)
- **frequently expose ourselves to destructive, chaotic influences**

Polar thinking

Our reality emerged as a process of creation from inseparable unity. We live in a *world of polarities*, between whose extremes we oscillate but never reach. As long as both sides alternate, as long as our life is in flow, we remain healthy.

Any kind of *stagnation* prevents this and lets the problem responsible for it sinks to a deeper level of materiality. It then materialises as a focus of disease.

The lack

Being arises through non-being, says a Far Eastern wisdom. Only by separating unity into polarities can materiality manifest itself. If the poles are brought together again, reality dissolves.

The visible is thus created through asymmetry. But this does not at the same time mean loss of harmony (= balancing of all polar opposites). Disharmony and thus also illness always point to a *deficiency*, to what is not lived. Symptoms occur because deficiencies prevail on one (or more) of the three levels: spirit-soul-body.

Processuality

Life-supporting Medicine is oriented towards

dynamic life processes
basic principles of the cosmos
asymmetries on the 3 levels spirit-soul-body

The focus is on the ***processuality*** of being, the constant change, the continuous transformation, which makes life possible in the first place. The fact that life was created at all must have a meaning, because nothing is meaningless (without spirit) in the universe. Just as everything is subject to a constant higher development, which we call evolution, our consciousness should also expand more and more. The experience necessary for this can only be gained in ***asymmetry***, not in the balancing of opposites. This deviation from the centre must not be static, but should be experienced alternately, and only as far as our constitution allows. Any persistence on one side (stagnation) has disease value (compare "Symmetropathy").

Illness expresses stagnation, shows standstill in personal development, whereby lack arises and can only be overcome by a higher development of consciousness, but without neglecting the material reality.

Substance or information – using the example of heavy metals

Whether at congresses or in the literature, contradictory statements about the effects of heavy metals, their diagnosis and therapy can be found again and again.

Amalgam is still on (almost) everyone's lips, which is why I would like to use this example to show the principle of the interaction of man and information and what causes the different ways of looking at things.

Mercury, which is present in a certain percentage in amalgam, belongs to the heavy metals. This classification concerns first of all the high weight, but can also be used in a figurative sense. Mercurius forms organic compounds that are difficult to dissolve, especially in combination with fat, and therefore poses a greater problem for detoxification. The half-life in the brain is 18 years!

Since high levels of stress can lead to neurological deficits, even personality changes, the concern of many doctors is understandably a thorough and lasting detoxification.

The methods that are used for this differ considerably – from purely material (e.g. Dimaval) to orthomolecular (selenium, zinc, vit. C) to purely informative (LSIT), everything is represented. What is striking is the broad spectrum of possibilities. Actually, there should be only one that is considered the best. This is obviously due to the different philosophies behind it, or to differences in quality that cannot yet be sufficiently objectified.

What is better, what is worse, what should be avoided, what has no effect?

In order to be able to answer these questions, some basic considerations are necessary. In the field of heavy metals, as hardly in any other consideration, we directly encounter the two world views that today – often without noticing it – are applied in parallel by one and the same person.

According to the old mechanistic world view, which has strongly influenced our medicine, mercury is a villain, which – comparable to microbes – is put down as the "cause" of diseases from a linear way of thinking. Experience shows, however, that neither the microbe nor a heavy metal necessarily leads to symptoms, but that there is obviously an *interaction* between the patient and its agent, which is highly individual and, due to the current cultural ignorance of people and science, usually results in a disease. Nevertheless, there are countless examples of people who do not fall ill in any way when exposed to comparable levels of stress. In the extreme, this is even a phenomenon known from the example of the poison cup or consumption of poisonous mushrooms. In correspondingly mentally mature people, no death effect occurs as a result.

There is no doubt that mercury is highly toxic and even life-threatening above a certain dose. However, we are talking here about doses that are at the limit or a few factors below it.

If we want to come to a better understanding of such seemingly contradicttory phenomena, we have to take a closer look at the interaction between substance and living organism.

First of all, we quickly realise that in living organisms, apart from a few mostly more mechanically conditioned links, there are no linear cause-effect relationships to be found.

In the meantime, however, we also know how two substances can interact with each other, once *mechanically*, but also through fields (field coupling) and finally also through *information exchange*. The latter is unusual because until now we have hardly any technologies that show us this as well as what we can constantly observe in the chemical-mechanical field in daily life. The interaction through information exchange has something to do with entropy, but also with further natural phenomena, where we are now just beginning to explore it properly and fundamentally.

However, the first two modes of action through mechanics and chemistry have in the meantime led to the unification, since both are actually only physics, which led to *field physics*, from which quantum physics emerged. From this point of view, the concept of matter has also changed.

Matter is not only mass, *but above all* energy & information.

However, information is involved in several ways, and there is much to suggest that there are different qualities of information. One is that which characterises the "particle of matter" (and can be described in mathematical formulae), another is that which characterises a kind of temporary state of being, thus linking past with future.

Material reality comes into being through the imprinting of a certain information.

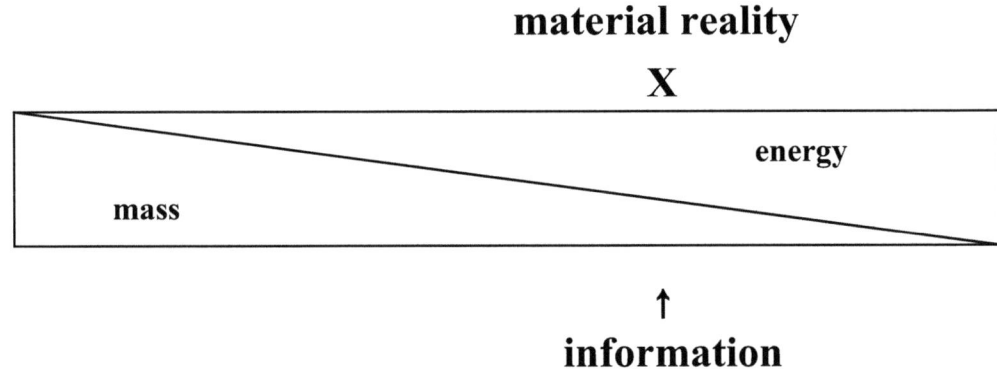

Fig. 31: The trinity of matter: mass – energy – information

If we look at symptoms produced by heavy metal exposure from this perspective, the first question is: "What information does this heavy metal contain?"

Since, as I said, it is a *heavy* metal, we next look at the mass. This yields a surprise: the actual mass of *every* matter (especially elementary particles) is a *natural constant*.

The mass density of e.g. mercury in relation to the "volume of space apparently occupied by the atom" is only 0.00000001 %! The "rest" of 99.9999999 % is vacuum, a massless "empty" space filled with virtual fluctuations. The (apparent) impenetrability and solidity of matter is achieved solely through the rotation movement and thus the fields of the particles.

Surprisingly, we thus realise that metals are only so (differently) hard because their inner characters are so different. Mercury is even liquid, although in the periodic table neighbouring metals are hard. Mercury is so completely different in the way it reacts and interacts with the other elements, although it has the same building blocks as water or gold. Only their internal arrangement, caused by information and the interaction make it total different to other substances.

In many respects, we live in an illusory world. The superficially visible matter is the expression of a spirit working in secret (which the Nobel Prize winner in physics Max Planck and the mathematician B. Riemann also postulated at the time in other physical contexts), which shapes the objects of existence through a wealth of specific information, especially the atoms and elementary particles.

To an even greater extent, we observe the effects of information in living complex systems, which are also not surprising, because there are no technical instruments or machines that can do without inner information. On the contrary – the more information we put into it, the more effective and useful it becomes.
So how much more must information be anchored and effective in living systems! It would be naïve to think that the technical information we know so far would be sufficient to keep such complex systems as "life" alive.

One is inevitably led to the insight that *effects* can only occur in the organism if the required information is present and is constantly adapted (adapted) in a highly intelligent way. We can even measure this to some extent! However, we are constantly exposed to innumerable pieces of information without any reactions.

So what is it that causes our organism to react in individual cases? It is the *resonance.* Only that information will cause a change to which we (or the biosystem of other living beings) go into resonance because it sees a necessity for it. We only draw in what is useful for our current overall situation. The prerequisite for this is conformity with already existing information, i.e. affinity to the status quo (transmitter-receptor-acceptor principle, cf. homeopathy).

If we resonate with mercury, there must be something in us that corresponds to it! If you look at the homeopathic remedy picture of Mercurius, you will notice that the "mercurial", the chaotic dominates with all the facets that an individual human being can offer. We can directly deduce from this that only those people will show effects who carry parts of it in themselves. However, very many do.

There is another agreement that corroborates this. In its effect on cell metabolism, mercury (which initially has an anabolic effect) can clearly be classified as catabolic (counter-regulation). The **catabolic metabolism** regulates the release of energy, but at the same time represents the unbridled chaotic part in us (correlates with right brain). To restore balance, **anabolic activity** would have to be increased. This means structure and order, but also **rhythm.**

We can encounter "good" and "bad" eliminators in practice. Some collect and retain, others release again quickly without burdening the organism in any way. The question of detoxification capacity is answered by the level of cell potential. Only at a normal value of -70 to -90 mV does the cell metabolism reach its extremely high performance of 30,000 – 100,000 chemical reactions/cell/second. These are only partly metabolic processes. In our polluted environment, they are increasingly detoxification functions. As a consolation, this capacity is far from being exhausted (Prof. Clausen). The prerequisite, however, is a normal cell potential. Detoxification is a catabolic process that takes place with <u>simultaneous</u> anabolic activity (ATP synthesis). Any disturbance of this equilibrium can impair the detoxification process. Wrong nutrition and psychological stress are at the top of the list.

Hardly known is the fact that the detoxification performance of the organism is directly dependent on the fat metabolism. The high energy expenditure necessary for detoxification cannot be covered by food alone (via ATP). For this purpose, a second pathway is used to cover up to 2/3 of the organism's energy needs. This is the absorption of long-wave components of sunlight by the π-electrons of unsaturated fats (linoleic and linolenic acid), especially in the skin. Electrons are known to interact with photons leading to excited states. These highly reactive fats also have a high autoxidation potential, which is why they magically attract oxygen.

Saturated fats can no longer participate in oxygen exchange because they have lost their free electrons. Inside the cell, they lead to cell death by asphyxiation; outside, they form clumps that are difficult to dissolve and lead to stasis in the lymphatic drainage. Mercury is highly lipophilic and therefore preferentially accumulates in fatty structures (cell membranes). If mercury also binds to the external fat deposits, the transit route of the matrix can be permanently blocked. Thus, it is at all understandable that mercury is also deposited in the water-containing connective tissue.

Interestingly, the dissolution of such complexes can occur through photo-chemical reactions, via excited states up to triplets (singlet states), through the supply of light of certain wavelengths, i.e. colours. The decay and dissolution of these complexes occurs. However, a sufficient number of unsaturated fats must still be present, or the redox and glutathione system must be functional. This photodynamic process is quite astonishing because of its apparent ease.

Here we see a comprehensible double effect of colours. The *mental* compo-nent is undisputed. Everyone reacts to it in a very individual way. The penetrating *material* effect of colours is again a well-known effect in chemistry. Now the almost philosophical question arises:

Can matter dissolve through the direct effect of the colours or through a change in the mental component?

If frequency jumps occur (octave shifting, constructive interference), the prerequisite for this is created by labilising the structure.

What can be derived from these findings of such an expanded world view for heavy metal pollution?

   - Whoever resonates with the characteristics of a heavy metal, with its information, will show symptoms with a tendency to deteriorate.

   - Those who are in a catabolic metabolic state will react more strongly to heavy metals (especially with neurological symptoms).

   - Those who are outside the cosmic order and thus lack rhythmicity will lose their health potential and thus their ability to detoxify.

Coincidences and lack of plan cannot exist in the universe, everything runs according to law. Every confrontation with any event in life, even if it is unpleasant, has a deeper meaning and should trigger something in us. By solving problems, we free ourselves from an unredeemed part of ourselves and come closer to salvation.

This epistemologically decisive contemplation is necessary in order to come to a new perspective. Otherwise, a renewal of our world and of medicine is inconceivable.

But now to **therapy:** The forcible, i.e. in principle chemical removal of a "mass", is a feasible way, but generally does not do justice to the problem. Side effects, for example from DMPS, are almost unavoidable.

However, if we see a heavy metal under the aspect of an intelligently ordered universe, then we suddenly understand what chance lies in this confrontation and *stop fighting*. Material reality only arises as polarity. When the polar extremes are balanced, neutrality prevails. There is then no danger for us.

Only when we leave symmetry, only in ASYMMETRY, can we gain experience and advance the formation of consciousness.

Heavy metal stress means asymmetry. High pollution means strong asymmetry. Only by *neutralising the heavy metal information* can we free ourselves from it. To do this, of course, we would have to know what the polar extreme to mercury is and, above all, what it *means.*

From a purely material point of view, the antidote could be given, possibly even titrated, in order to work as precisely as possible. However, this only works theoretically because mercury is not present in pure form but bound to salts. It works much better on the mental track.

In the end, it is always the LACK that separates us from unity, from salvation.

This way of thinking, which may well cause some readers to feel alienated, points to the real paradigm shift that will take place not only in science but also in medicine. The primary aim is not to establish a new system of science, but to awaken a new *awareness* of the inner connections of reality, thereby deepening and supplementing the understanding of existing scientific components. Through the expected successes, the whole of science will follow suit of its own accord.

It is therefore a matter of recognising and using the *all-unity consciousness*, which we should first and foremost anchor in ourselves, as a powerful active principle – in medicine for the benefit of patients! Only when we as pioneers, as therapists, live and act in this consciousness every day, then we can act successfully externally – in the treatment of our patients as well as in our encounters with other people.

Everything that is thought and done in the All-Unity Consciousness happens, and happens instantaneously. Nothing then separates us from the divine spirit, the primordial informant of all things.

Whoever takes this step of realisation will find peace. All fighting gradually ceases, because there is no longer any confrontation with "enemies", or any confrontation is handed over to the instance of truth and justice, whereby the attacker then has to deal with the totality of creation and no longer with the individual, the attacked. Every "attack" will be understood as a message, as a signal for renewal, which in this way will finally begin and, if practised correctly, will also take place. Nothing happens by chance in the universe. Behind everything there is a higher meaning, an absolute justice, the divine mathematics of life and being!

Trouble results from the impatience and unwillingness to take things as they "really" are. Some message is unpleasant for us only because it reminds us deep down of an unredeemed conflict. The "negative" therefore lies hidden, unrecognised or unconscious within ourselves until we are compelled by insight or external "realities" (what we call fate) to finally resolve it.

A therapist can only really treat successfully if he is at peace with himself. From a higher consciousness, he can understand the patient as a building block in God's plan, which, as the healing process progresses, also allows something in himself to become whole.

Healing "happens" when there is a willingness to change and the patient himself strives for the renewal of the cosmic order, which is predetermined by the spiritual laws.

In summary, it can be said that heavy metal pollution is also a soul-spiritual problem that needs to be solved. The confrontation with an agent does not happen by chance, but obeys spiritual laws like everything in the universe.

The "message" contained in it should be taken up and implemented. Necessary processes of consciousness can thus be set in motion. With appropriate therapeutic help, the patient can be enabled to recognise and compensate for his deficiency. War becomes peace, fighting becomes love and understanding. Thus the patient automatically transforms his originally wrong resonance to things, thoughts, deeds, into a new, higher, more correct resonance. His burden disappears and he becomes symptom-free in the end. The heavy metal can then be eliminated without any problem – guided by the inherent intelligence of the body and soul – via the excretory organs. (This chapter was co-authored by Prof. Dr. E. Kaucher).

Diagnostics in Life-supporting Medicine

Diagnosis is based on 3 pillars:

Psychological correlate of the disease
Reasons for the metabolic derailment
Permanent stresses on the mesenchyme

This threefold division reflects a *holographic pattern* that can be found everywhere. If one looks at the whole organism, the tripartite division is the same as at organ or cell level. *Consciousness* is found at all levels of being.

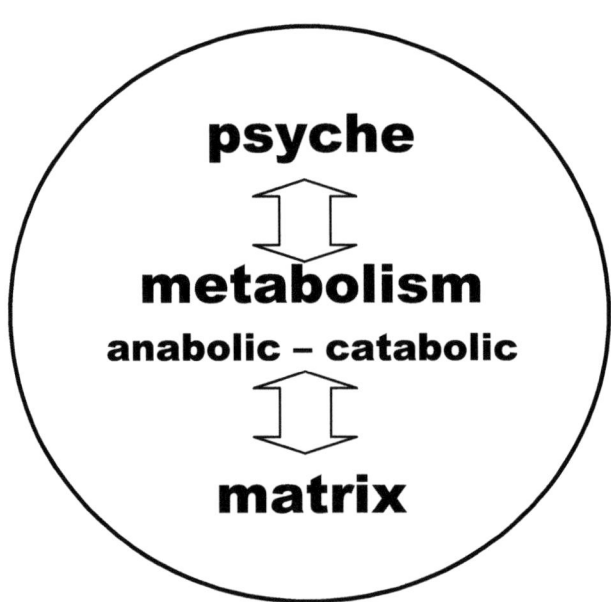

Fig. 32: The interaction of the 3 areas of the organism

The aim is always to work out the stressful information on all levels of being in order to get behind the "idea" of the illness.

Access to the **psyche** is found through various test procedures – from the Luescher test to Psychokinesiology and Neurolistic Programming NLP. The following questions are of primary interest:

- **What is not in conformity with life?**
- **What life lie is behind the illness?**
- **What is rejected and therefore not lived?**
- **What longings are there, where is the lack?**
- **What disturbs the cosmic order?**
- **Which spiritual laws are permanently violated?**
- **Through what is the primordial trust undermined?**
- **What kind of false consciousness prevents the necessary reorientation?**

The **metabolic derailment** is verified by bio-energetic measuring methods as well as blood-hormone analyses. Here it is especially important to recognise *latent insufficiencies of the endocrine glands* that only appear under stress. Very often, *dysthyroidism* is overlooked because the morning blood test in a rested state cannot tell us anything about the demands of everyday life to which the patient is exposed. Metabolic rigidity may have its possible cause here.

Likewise, the function of the adrenal glands must be checked, preferably by stress tests.

The changes in the **matrix** can also be determined by bioenergetic tests or by blood analyses, as well as imaging procedures (cf. Chapter "Systematic Procedure" at the end).

Therapy in Life-supporting Medicine
The *therapy* is based on the results of the diagnosis and means:

Transformation into life-supporting information

This refers to all conditions in life that are not life-conforming – on all three levels. The pure life energy, the bioplasm (the Qi of the Chinese) may have absorbed foreign information in the course of time through various events and thus have become *contaminated.* Healing can only occur when the patient frees himself from this (or with help from outside). However, *information* cannot be dissolved into thin air, but only transformed into a more complex one. This should be of higher value compared to the previous one and thus more attractive (new attractor).

The 3 main questions that have to be solved through therapy are:

1) How can the psychological correlate underlying the illness be transformed?
2) How can the metabolic derailment be normalised?
3) How can the mesenchyme are freed from stress, the degree of order be increased and the balance of juices be normalised?

The additional question should be:

How can rhythm (= flexibility, adaptability, regulation) **be restored on all 3 levels?**

This fulfils the universally valid *3 + 1 rule*, which is indispensable for a holistic approach.

The key to the solution on the *soul-spiritual level* lies in

Strict adherence to spiritual laws
Conflict resolution through forgiving and forgiveness
Integration of unlived aspects (shadows)

The key to the *metabolic-regulatory level* lies in

Consistent change of diet
Normal function of the endocrine glands
Counterpolar treatment (anabolic or catabolic)

The key for the *mesenchyme level* lies in

Elimination of toxins and waste products
Acid-base balance & charge carriers (fats)
Support of redox and glutathione systems

The *general key* for all levels lies in the restoration of the

Rhythm of regulation-counter-regulation

As this extremely important aspect of rhythmics receives very little attention in medicine, a few remarks on this (cf. Chapter 2). According to H. Heine, the homeostasis of the tissue is established by rhythms. Rhythm means movement, adaptation, flexibility. It counteracts stagnation and is therefore essential for the flow of life.

Rhythm, however, also means order, as fixed, pre-programmed sequences are thus called up. The biorhythms are synchronised by external cosmic rhythms. This shows the integration of the human being into the universal laws of the cosmos. This knowledge should therefore be a central component of every therapy.

The body cells are integrated into a strict hierarchy that is controlled by the brain. However, they have a high degree of autonomy that enables them to maintain everyday metabolism. (For example, they build up and dismantle their receptors independently.) They therefore have cell consciousness (which has been proven in many experiments) as well as the larger associations have their own organ consciousness (compare Chinese teaching of the 5 phases of transformation).

The body has a segmental structure (Mendeleev structures). These segments of the trunk have autonomy which is maintained as long as possible. Inflammations (and thus also pain) initially remain segmentally limited before they spread to neighbouring segments. The nervous system plays an essential role in symptom propagation (projection) (cf. Bergsmann). This is why there is also a strict energetic separation into left and right halves of the body from the neck region downwards. Peripheral foci can therefore only affect the same side centrally (e.g. the tooth region), not the opposite side.

A successful therapy must start at the level of organisation where the main problem lays – cellular level, organ level, or the whole organism. However, all 3 levels should always be addressed *simultaneously* – psyche, metabolic regulation, matrix.

Even if, for example, the psychological aspect is in the foreground, the other two levels should always be treated as well!

For the therapist, therefore, 3 + 1 questions arise after the diagnosis:

On which level is the main problem (deficiency)?

What can be done for the other two levels?
How can the necessary energy be provided?
+
How can the stagnation be rhythmically dissolved?

The secret for success is to use the therapy impulses *rhythmically on all three levels.* This means that after each stimulus the counter-regulation is waited for and even specifically supported. It should be noted that the impulse in the direction of balance, i.e. towards the individual centre, is always stronger than the one leading away from it.

The principle of stimulation or dampening in rhythmic sequence can be applied by all branches of medicine.

The principle should always be taken to heart to meet the patient where he or she is. This refers on the one hand to the communication and the level of understanding that can be chosen, but on the other hand to his condition.
A very weak patient requires a completely different approach than one who is still very fit. In both cases, however, there is a weakness in the energy balance, either localized, so that it can be compensated, or overarching, so that it is felt as languor.

If we want to transform disease-causing information, then this is always an active, energy-consuming process. For this reason, more or less intensive care should be taken to primarily improve the energy balance. This is not only a question of catabolic metabolic activity. The more advanced the disease, the more serious the damage on the material level in the area of the "body battery", the lipoproteids.

The basics of this were discussed in detail in chapter 2. However, before starting to supply highly unsaturated fatty acids in combination with proteins (as lipoproteids), it should be ensured that the multiple fat clumps (precipitates of hardened fat) in the mesenchyme can be broken down. In addition to the supply of enzymes, all lactic fermented vegetables (sauerkraut, beetroot, etc.) are suitable for this purpose and should be administered in relatively large quantities at the beginning. At the same time, important colourings (flavonoids), vitamins and minerals are supplied in this way.

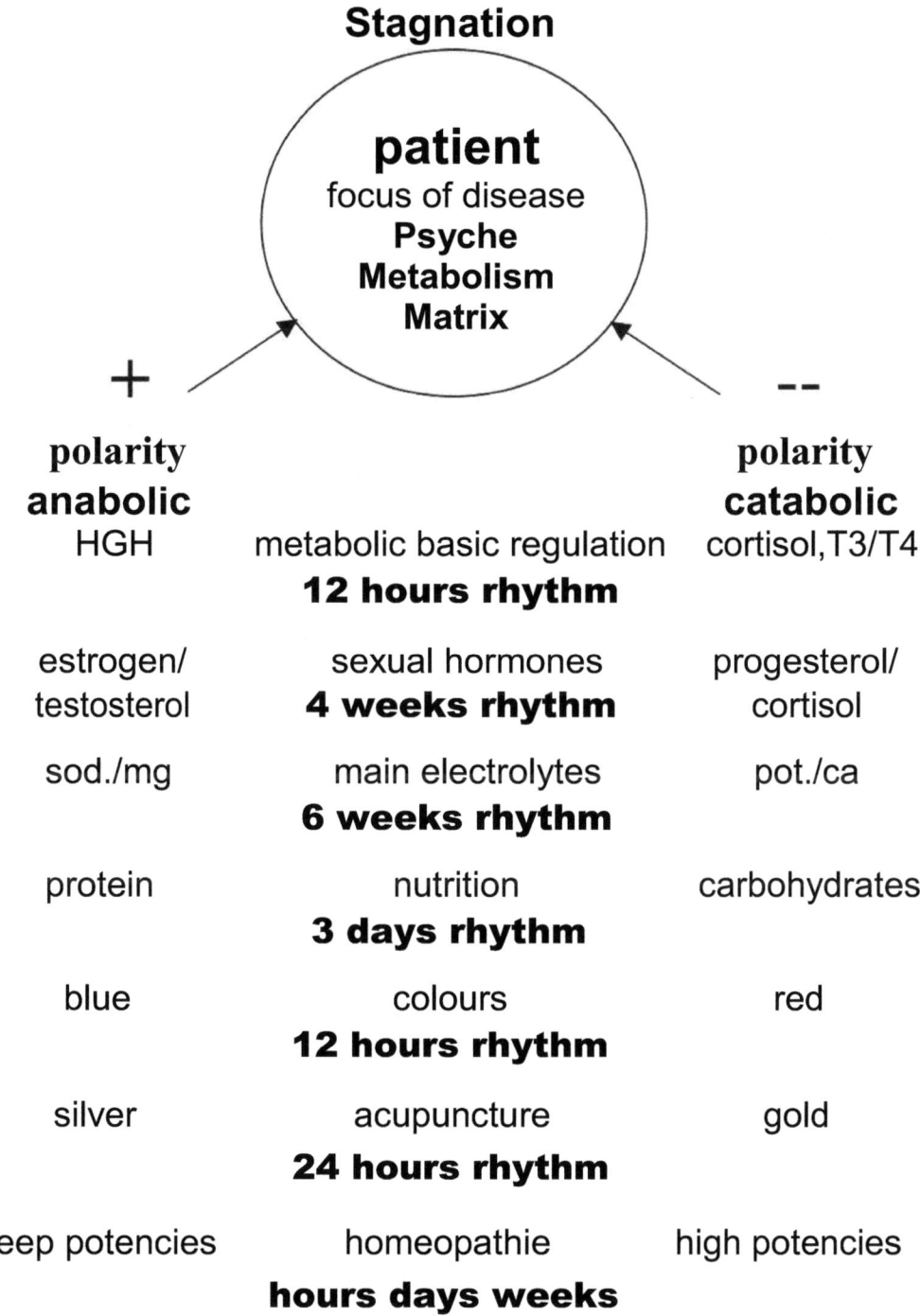

Fig. 33: Triggering regulation and counter-regulation through rhythms

The material basis for the absorption of energy from the light is created by the oil-protein diet. This can be intensified considerably in advanced cases (e.g. cancer) by linseed oil enemas of up to 250 ml daily. In addition, the tumour region can be rubbed with linseed oil for subsequent red light irradiation. This is possible in the practice with a special, water-cooled IR device or laser.

At home, it would be possible to use a commercially available red light lamp. For cooling, a large square vase filled with water is placed in front of it. This way, the distance to the lamp can be reduced considerably, which results in a much higher intensity. Homeopathic remedies can also be placed in the water, which are then transferred as informed light. The irradiation time can be several hours.

AM-Integ – the special therapy method

Even though the treatment method described here is mainly interesting for those therapists who use Living Systems Information Therapy (LSIT), it can give food for thought for similar procedures, as it is based on the quite natural principle of **grafting.**

Anyone who knows a little about trees and has experienced how a small branch from a noble tree, e.g. a blue spruce, is grafted onto an ordinary spruce, thus turning it into a beautiful blue spruce, will be amazed at how such a thing is possible. The reason lies hidden in a primal principle that prevails in nature: the higher (spiritual) order prevails.

As already explained in Chapter 2, the organism adopts external rhythms if they have a higher order. This is also evident at the cellular level.

From this and from the overall understanding of life-supporting medicine, which is based on the alchemistic principle separation – transformation – integration, the therapy method presented here was developed. It is assumed that it is a question of the dose whether a substance has an adverse or a healing effect (Hippocrates: "It's the dose that counts").

A more differentiated view of pollutants, but also usually of materials classified as "non-harmful" would be desirable in principle. After all, the small amount of a substance initially means an anabolic stimulus for metabolism and immune system, which forces a reaction. This does not have to mean elimination, but can mean integration – even in the case of harmful substances.

Epictate said: "It is not things that are bad, but how we think about them".

It is not mercury that is bad, but how we (and our organism) deal with it. An overload with it is very often associated with symptoms of illness – but only because the principle of life was not observed in advance. If we separate, the harmful can be separated from the useful, the former can be eliminated and the latter can be integrated. This can also be done retrospectively, when symptoms of illness have already occurred.

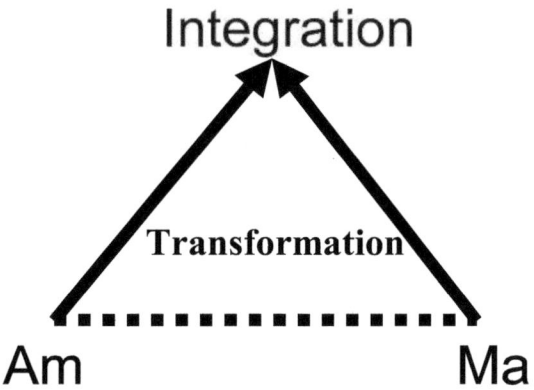

Legend:
A = **AGENT** total information *strong*
m = information „human" *weak*
M = HUMAN total information *strong*
a = information „agent" *weak*

The practice looks like this:
From the patient, the healthy total info is obtained by subtracting from the total organism the agent (electronically). This is the **M.**

From the disease focus, the info is extracted. This is the **A.**

Now the healthy total info "human" is contaminated with some info from the focus of the disease, at the same time the focus of the disease is informed (grafted) with some "healthy human being".

The healing formula is:

$$\text{AGENT} \times \textbf{Human} \qquad \text{human} \times \textbf{Agent}$$

The two healing information obtained in this way are transferred to carriers (physiological saline solution) and simultaneously applied internally (A x m), as well as externally (M x a), rhythmically 3 days/week and 4 days break. The effect is noticeable and resounding.

Therapist

Under no circumstances should a type of treatment be considered on its own, detached from the therapist. One should always be clear about this. Just as illness is a resonance issue, the healing process itself is resonant with what resonates in the therapist. The inner attitude towards the patient, the compassion (empathy – not pity!), the personal attention – the intention determine the success. Healing is always an active process that the patient has to accomplish himself. The necessary prerequisites for the therapist are

seeking one's centre
going into resonance
LOVE

LOVE means the all-embracing selfless love that should flow through the therapist, detached from the ego, in order to be able to give the patient entrusted to him the best possible help for his healing process.

Love means: **Understanding everything**
forgiving everything
no demands
nothing expected
only giving.

Novalis said, "Love is the Amen of the universe."

This can be compared to a lake into which one dives, can throw off all ballast and, in an indescribable lightness of being, experiences the grace of God as an all-pervading feeling of happiness.

You should let yourself be guided by your intuition (soul aspect) and inspiration (spirit aspect). Only then will optimal resonance be possible. Pecuniary considerations (which are definitely relevant for a practice leadership) should take a back seat. This means that all actions of the therapist and all his therapeutic considerations should be based on a *high sense of ethical responsibility.*

It is necessary that the therapist is fully aware of the *interaction* with the patient. Healing happens at the interpersonal level. It is therefore necessary to find the right attitude, comparable to a photo lens (focus)

intention
concentration
contemplation

This inner attitude means giving up the idea of doing in favour of being (right awareness).

Every person, especially a therapist should test the rightness of all their actions by two words: *How* and *Why*. These are the basic principles of ethics.

The "how" shows him with what attitude of mind he acts. Is he in his centre, or does he have problems of his own that he may be "passing on"? The "why" reveals which egoistic or altruistic intentions he is pursuing. It is very helpful to make this clear to oneself again and again. Those who are in cosmic harmony on both points are really acting in conformity with life.

Patient

Healing happens when the return to the cosmic order has taken place (religio). Health remains stable when the spiritual laws are observed. It is as simple as that (in principle). The reality is usually different, however, usually due to complete ignorance of the situation, *why* a person has become ill.

Therefore, there are 3 questions (3 x **W** according to A. Kriele) that the patient should answer:

What do you lack? (deficiency)
What do you want? (goal)
What can I do for you? (help)

The last question should be asked 6 times, each time with a different emphasis in the word order. This also implies the possibilities and *limits* that exist in practice. It points out, the responsibility remains with the patient. He can expect help, but not a cure.

It is a major concern of *Life-supporting Medicine* to provide *comprehensive patient education*. This concerns all circumstances that have led to an illness, but far beyond that also the possibilities of psychohygiene and all philosophical questions about the meaning of life and the expansion of consciousness through knowledge and thus also prevention.

It should become clear to the patient how an illness holds up a mirror to him and reveals deficits. Only he himself is in a position to put an end to the deficiency and to transform the stagnation in the asymmetry of his life back into a dynamic flow. He should therefore answer the burning question of what his deepest, hidden desires are, how he would shape his life if it were only up to him. Then he would perhaps come to know what his inner self had planned for this life and could – even if sometimes very late – still realise himself and find his life's task.

Of course, the patient should also be informed about the various treatment options as well as the methods. However, it is important to convey that these are only a means to an end, i.e. they do not "cure" themselves. To become healed, more is needed. First of all, the insight that not everyone else is "to blame" for one's suffering (victim role), but that the patient has shaped his or her own destiny. This is the only way to awaken the willingness to take the initiative. Only in this way can the willingness to take the initiative be awakened. Talks on this basis not only strengthen trust in the therapist, but are also an indispensable prerequisite for the full success of the therapy.

Furthermore, it should be made clear that every person has his or her own individual chance to become healthy. There is no single stage – no matter what the disease – in which healing is impossible (compare spontaneous healing in cancer). Although this contradicts conventional textbook medicine, it corresponds to experience. This means for us:

We must not make false promises of healing to patients that would be charlatanism. But we can show them the path that can lead them out of any situation (if they want to take it). This path is called self-discovery, back to the cosmic order.

The 9 principles of harmony, as advocated by the Breema therapists, can be helpful:

1) **Take part in everything you do – with body, feeling and thinking.**
2) **Always and everywhere make sure that your body is comfortable.**
3) **Do only one activity at a time.**
4) **Never use force at any time** (let flow).
5) **Always be true and act without judgement.**
6) **In each of your actions: Do not hurry, but do not hesitate either.**
7) **In all your actions: Be gentle and firm at the same time.**
8) **All living things support each other. Every moment you have the possibility to give as well as to receive.**
9) **Nothing special! To be who we really are, to express our true nature, nothing extra is necessary.**

It is not primarily a matter of finding the reasons why the patient has become ill – that is already in the past – but of finding the opportunities for reorientation and reshaping that will enable him to get out of this stuck situation of chronic illness, reasons that will reveal the lack.

In this process, his inner attitude and mindset has a very significant influence on the healing process. Nothing should be fought, but first and foremost *strengthened.* The patient should do everything to support his healthy cells and organs – mentally as well as materially. This includes a conscious diet and sufficient exercise as well as mental hygiene. It is important to observe the law of focus and blur: What I focus on becomes my reality (cf. Fig. 33).

If the reality is to be changed, if a focus of illness is to dissolve, then this can only be achieved by transformation and taking it out of focus. If the attention is directed to a certain area, it strengthens it.

The health potential is strengthened by all those measures that are in conformity with life.

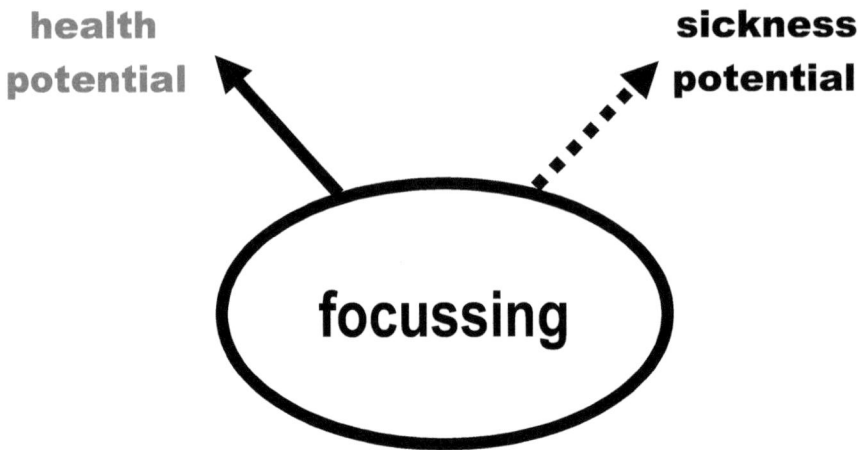

Fig. 34: Law of sharpness and blur – the viewer creates reality

Physical peculiarities

For a general understanding, it is important to point out some peculiarities of the organism. First of all, it is necessary to correctly classify the *function of the immune system*. Nothing runs in the organism without (at least) accompanying measures of defence. Even regeneration processes are not possible without phagocytosis (a catabolic process).

The immune system is dependent on all 3 areas and is subject to the

mental mood
metabolic state
condition of the matrix

From psychoneuroimmunology we know the different influences, from which the consequences for practice can be derived:

A fully functional immune system as the basis for an organism with integrity depends on the trouble-free interplay of all three levels of being and their rhythms.

Furthermore, it must be pointed out that our immune system only tries to rid itself of toxic burdens in the context of an acute illness – which should be understood as a healing reaction.

Already after 1 week it usually stops its efforts and *comes to terms with its burdens.* There is then a stady state in the organism between *permanent stress* and the immune system. Only by setting an *attention signal* (domain of LSIT) can detoxification processes be activated.

Summary

Life-supporting Medicine is oriented towards all aspects that are necessary for the preservation of life and health. Any kind of fighting "against something" is alien to it. Therefore, it is not the intention to oust conventional medicine from its territory. Rather, it is about pointing out new viable paths that all therapists can follow, no matter what direction they come from.

What has been missing so far – and this is the main shortcoming – has been a coherent, overarching concept that unites all directions in medicine under one umbrella. Therefore, the first priority is the idea of unity. To achieve this, an important step has to be taken – from semantics to syntactics. This will ultimately lead to a **Unified Medicine**. The foundations for this have been laid out in the author's new "Textbook for the UNITED life-supporting MEDICINE", published by the same publishing house.

If it is assumed that everything in the entire universe is linked to everything else, then every impulse will necessarily be able to reach every place. However, reactions only apear when **resonance** occurs, i.e. when the information of the impulse is similar or the same as that of the receiver. Therefore, everything we send out, every impulse – triggered by actions, words or thoughts – also comes back to us.

Reality is therefore a mirror of our actions. But we also have it in our hands to change reality at any time, even to conquer serious illnesses.

The entire universe obeys the law of polarity. All being presents itself in 2 extremes, which appear neutral overall. Only by leaving the middle, by the resulting asymmetry, do tensions arise, but these are the root for experience and thus knowledge. However, it is important not to live one-sidedly, but in an alternating passage through the polar aspects of reality. Only this **processsuality of BEING**, the constant transformation of the present, the stream of life. Every **stagnation in an asymmetry** has a high disease value because it leads to a **lack**. Every symptom of illness arises from a deficit that may have arisen on the various levels. However, the starting point is always the information contained in an idea. Only through constant repetition of the information (iteration), which results from one-sidedness, from stagnation, does the materialisation of this thought quantum field structure occur, which we then call the focus of disease.

It is therefore a question of each person's **consciousness** whether they recognise these connections, accept their personal situation as "home-made" and are ready for change, for **transformation into life-supporting information**. Only in this way can the life energy unfold freely, can burden some contaminations be removed and all necessary information flow freely again. For the organism this means: the restoration of a **dynamic order** through **rhythm** and **sound.**

In order to proceed efficiently, a 3-point diagnosis should be made, which is oriented towards the focal points of **psyche – metabolism – matrix**. Derived from this, the therapy concept is also created according to 3 points. All 3 levels are always treated, but with different weighting. The treatment aims to **transform** what is already there and also to restore **rhythms**. Thus the universal 3+1 rule is fulfilled.

The treatment can be carried out with the various possibilities that a practice has to offer. All areas of medicine can be integrated, including conventional medical methods.

Through the use of new **energetic therapy methods**, both diagnostics and therapy can be made much simpler and more efficient. Nevertheless, the material basis must not be forgotten, which primarily concerns nutrition. It must be ensured that the energy balance improves and that the patients can quickly implement the healing information.

The therapist's commitment, qualification and high ethical responsibility are decisive for the success of the therapy.

Life-supporting Medicine is not (yet) taught at university. Doctors who feel called to offer their patients an optimum of treatment can be trained according to this methodology. By successfully completing this further training, they can be accepted into a pool of highly qualified therapists. Modern means of communication are used for optimisation. In the future, they will have access to diagnostic centres with high-tech equipment via a **network** and will also be connected to each other, which will further increase the effectiveness of their work and create the best conditions for highly effective, yet *cost-effective* medicine. This then also enables adequate remuneration for high qualified performance, which ensures the financial security of the practice.

By frequently dispensing with expensive imaging procedures or elaborate laboratory tests, costs can be drastically reduced, even if more effort is required initially. The difference between this and allopathic therapy, however, is that with each life-supporting measure, through each treatment step, the patient's health potential is raised, which drastically reduces susceptibility to future illness. The goal on the physical level is therefore to restore self-regulation to such an extent that the autonomous life processes can once again run undisturbed.

Patients are actively involved in the healing process and retain responsibility towards their bodies and life. This requires comprehensive education in all areas.

Patients interested in Life-supporting Medicine have access to doctors' addresses via the Internet and, in future, via a central call box.

On a *physical level*, all treatments have the goal of achieving a higher dynamic degree of order. An indispensable prerequisite for this is a deep inner peace. Only on this can a high dynamic be built up. This requires trust in the therapist and his methods, but also unshakeable trust in the higher divine guidance, which is unfortunately lacking in most people today.

In the beginning, only weak stimuli should be given, and then gradually increased. Rhythms should be observed (e.g. 1x/week on a certain day and at the same time).

The procedure in practice is summarised again here.

▶ According to the rules of life-supporting Medicine, diagnosis and therapy are always carried out on **3 levels** – psyche, metabolic regulation, matrix. Depending on how serious the problem is, other areas can be added. The basis is always nutrition.

▶ Every *chronically ill* patient is examined in the practice to see whether they are suffering from an *anabolic or catabolic* disease and how far their **metabolism** deviates from the norm. At the same time, the reaction to stress is tested (regulation). This can be done in a very time-saving bioenergetic way with the VEGA-SRT, ZMR 703 or the new MORA*nova*. The determination of the "Total Anabolic Activity" (TAA) is more complex. It is essential to ensure that the adrenal gland and thyroid gland are functioning properly, otherwise substitution is necessary!

▶ Increased attention is paid to the **catabolic *heat-energy balance*** and the degree of hyperacidity. Both correlate with the functionality of the fat structures (lipoproteids) and thus the number of free electrons. Heavy metal pollution or other environmental toxins, electrosensitivity as well as chronic fatigue are indicative of a disturbance in the area of fats.

▶ Similarly, **anabolic *inflammations*** are in focus. They lead to a loss of order, which at the same time worsens the transmission of information as well as the direct absorption of energy from sunlight. All measures that relieve the matrix, the supply of lipoproteins through food (combined with sunlight), as well as therapeutic tones and sounds are suitable to raise the dynamic degree of order in the tissue again.

▶ The question always arises as to what the patient is *lacking*, what makes it impossible for him to accomplish normal metabolic regulation. The search has to take place *on all levels of being*, whereby the new ordering system – the Luescher life cube – is a decisive help. From the working diagram (page 121) it can be seen where and why the metabolic regulation may be disturbed, which results in a direct therapeutic approach.

▶ *All* therapeutic approaches must always be examined to see whether they are suitable for normalising the *blocked part*. For catabolic diseases such as CHD or cancer, all measures should be *anabolically* effective and vice versa. The goal is always to strengthen the weaker portion, but not to take away a "too much".

▶ The "how" should dominate over the "what". Every loving attention promotes the healing process, every "administration" inhibits it. The *intention* of the practitioner decisively shapes the therapy outcome. Therefore, the exact knowledge about the physiological processes is very crucial. Any stasis or stagnation must be brought back into the flow of life. Whether this is done in a deep material way or in the psyche – every level should always be treated.

▶ The healing process does not happen passively from the outside (through the therapist), but means active cooperation of the patient. The more he is involved in the responsibility, the more intensively the necessary processes of consciousness can take place.

► The success of the treatment can be recognised directly by measuring the metabolism, which is also suitable for monitoring the course of the treatment, optimising the dose, monitoring the diet, prophylaxis against relapses, etc. This gives the doctor much more certainty in the assessment and therapy of chronically ill patients. Each treatment method can thus be tested for its effectiveness itself, which saves a lot of time that is often lost through "trial and error".

► No treatment should take place without specific nutritional recommend-dations. This is the basis and promotes the patients' awareness of their body. The rhythm should be observed. The focus should be on gaining quality of life, because that is the best motivation.

Concluding remarks

For naturopathically oriented doctors, knowledge of the basic regulation system according to Pischinger is obligatory. Unfortunately, the "freestyle", namely dealing with the basics of metabolic regulation, is usually no longer part of the programme, nor is the fundamental knowledge of fat metabolism. But anyone who has dealt with this intensively can hardly imagine ever treating their patients again without this basic knowledge.

What is the special value for the practice?
Medicine could be much simpler, more manageable and more efficient, especially with the large number of chronic diseases. In my opinion, the high number of chronic diseases is not primarily due to increasing environ-mental stress, but to a misunderstanding of pathophysiological processes in the organism. Linear causal thinking quickly leads to the limits of what is possible. Complex networked structures, such as the organism has, cannot be comprehensively analysed from the outside. Therefore, it is necessary to work out the simple (!) basic principles on which functional processes are based.

Synthesis *is the name of the new path that will make medicine successful again.*

All processes taking place in the organism and every emotional expression are inseparably linked to the metabolic regulation of the cells. All diagnostic and therapeutic considerations must therefore take their laws into account. However, these are clearly manageable, as they are subject to a polar prin-ciple. After the current situation of the cell metabolism as well as the basic psycho-energetic structure of the individual patient has been determined and classified in the Luescher life cube, all therapeutic measures are derived from this – from medication to nutrition. But also the progress of the therapy can be read from the changed metabolic situation, which creates an enormous therapy security.

The basis for a correct understanding is provided by the **three-component theory** according to J. Schole, as well as **psychoenergetics** according to Luescher. Anyone who has familiarised himself with these overarching theories and applies them in his practice will hardly be able to imagine practising medicine without this knowledge before. The success with his chronically ill patients underlines this in a lasting way.

However, the normalisation of metabolic regulation can only take place when four things are guaranteed:

1) The energy uptake must be normalised via the lipoproteids.
2) The psychodurable stress is dissolved
3) The matrix freed from its serious stresses
4) The liquid balance and composition must be equalized.

This does not happen without consciousness processes. For this, the psyche must give the "green light", through the regained readiness for transformation and change. Every stagnation, every rejection of certain aspects of life, every unresolved conflict prevents this in the long term. Only a transformed consciousness is capable of this.

A successful treatment brings the patient forward in his spiritual development, which has repercussions for the therapist. With the patient's is being healed, something in him or herself also becomes healed. When this happens, which is a grace from God, we have reaped the real reward for our work.

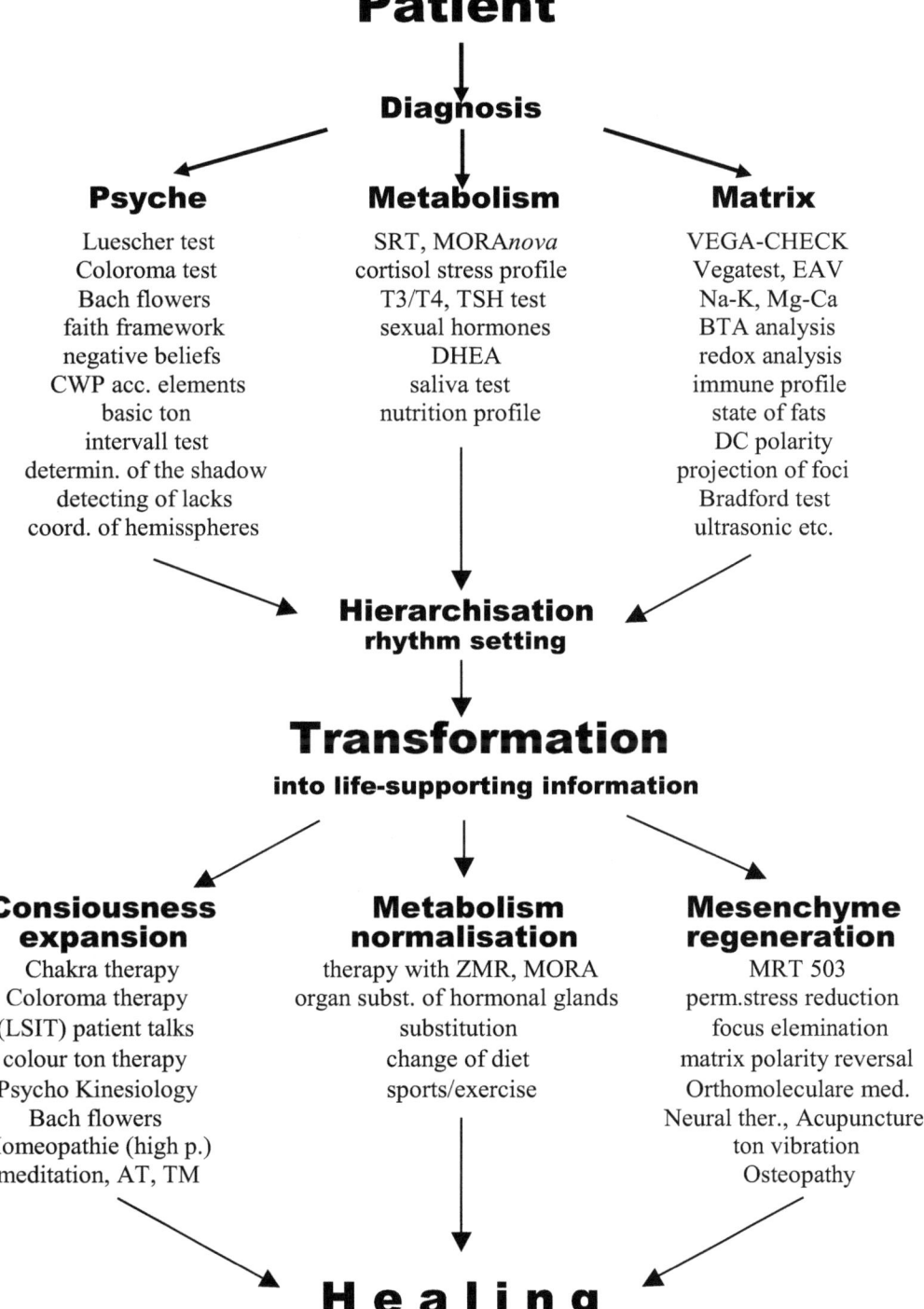

Patient

↓

Diagnosis

Psyche   **Metabolism**   **Matrix**

Psyche	Metabolism	Matrix
Luescher test	SRT, MORA*nova*	VEGA-CHECK
Coloroma test	cortisol stress profile	Vegatest, EAV
Bach flowers	T3/T4, TSH test	Na-K, Mg-Ca
faith framework	sexual hormones	BTA analysis
negative beliefs	DHEA	redox analysis
CWP acc. elements	saliva test	immune profile
basic ton	nutrition profile	state of fats
intervall test		DC polarity
determin. of the shadow		projection of foci
detecting of lacks		Bradford test
coord. of hemisspheres		ultrasonic etc.

Hierarchisation
rhythm setting

↓

Transformation
into life-supporting information

Consiousness   **Metabolism**   **Mesenchyme**
expansion   **normalisation**   **regeneration**

Consiousness expansion	Metabolism normalisation	Mesenchyme regeneration
Chakra therapy	therapy with ZMR, MORA	MRT 503
Coloroma therapy	organ subst. of hormonal glands	perm.stress reduction
(LSIT) patient talks	substitution	focus elemination
colour ton therapy	change of diet	matrix polarity reversal
Psycho Kinesiology	sports/exercise	Orthomoleculare med.
Bach flowers		Neural ther., Acupuncture
Homeopathie (high p.)		ton vibration
meditation, AT, TM		Osteopathy

Healing

8. Learning aids

Health

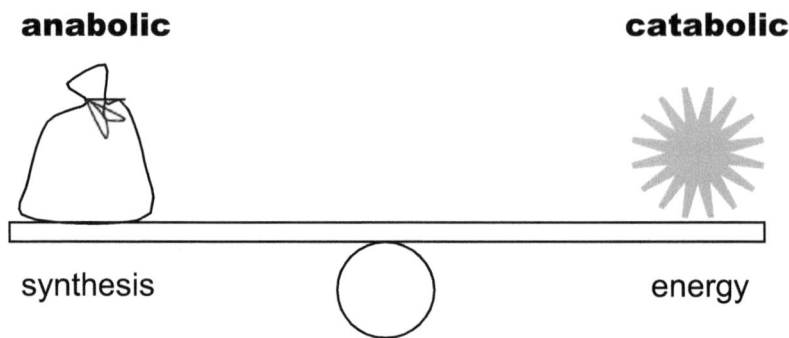

anabolic   **catabolic**

synthesis   energy

Step 1: diagnostical considerations
Capture the *idea of the sickness* – where is the lack?

chronic disease

anabolic   catabolic ???

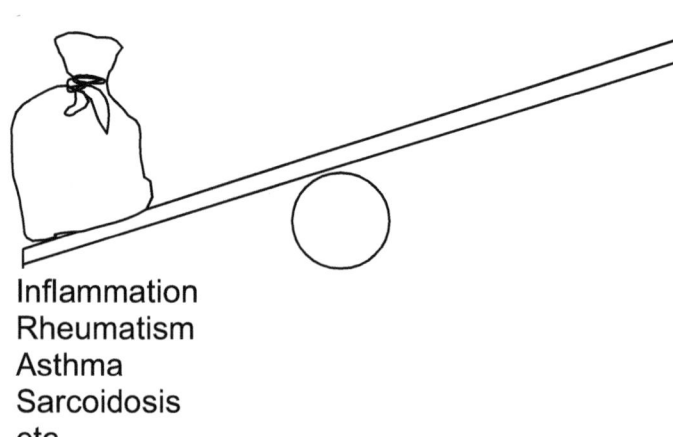

Inflammation
Rheumatism
Asthma
Sarcoidosis
etc.

3 points:

- ◆ **Psychic correlate of sickness** (conflicts)
- ◆ **Metabolic derailment** (kind and reasons)
- ◆ **Changes of the matrix** (burdens, liquid balance)

Step 2: Work out the psychic correlate

- o primal trauma
- o unresolved conflict
- o negative beliefs
- o religious belief system
- o life theme, rejected parts (shadow)
- o constitutional weakness (5 phases of change)
- o **Luescher test (columns)**

Step 3: Determine the metabolic state

- o measure with SRT, ZMR, MORA*nova* or blood test
- o compare with typical symptoms:

anabolic	catabolic
(decreased catabolic activity)	**(decreased anabolic activity)**
- tiredness	- restlessness, nervousness
- feeling of heaviness	- night sweats
- susceptibility to infections	- hot soles (at night)
- lack of concentration	- sleep disturbances
- listlessness	- inner heat
- slow movement and speech	- thirst, dry mouth
- anxiety, resignation	- jumpiness
- feeling of fullness, flatulence	- fast, hasty speech
- no recovery through sleep	- susceptibility to stress
- frequent freezing, cold limbs	- tendency to anger
- water retention	- little reserves
- aversion to cold food	- dizziness
- frigidity or impotence	- headaches
- menstrual disorders	- weight problems ($\uparrow$ or $\downarrow$)

Step 4: Placement in the Luescher cube

Preparation:
  1) determine columns by Luescher test
  2) measure metabolic state

Assignment:
  1) locate corner of preferred colour (++)
  2) compare measured metabolic state
  3) find the corner of the rejected colour (- -)
  4) draw a connecting line

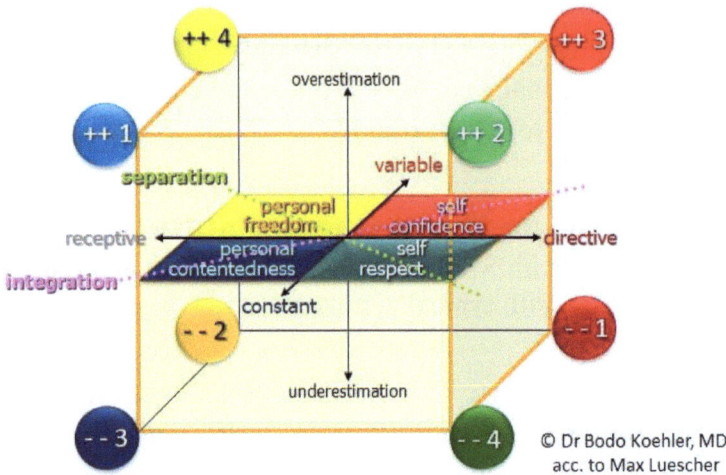

© Dr Bodo Koehler, MD
acc. to Max Luescher

Evaluation:
  1) current symptoms (= compensation)
    - acute anabolic or catabolic?
    - which hormonal regulator is active?
    - which mineral is in excess?
    - which food harms?
    - which psychostructure dominates?

  2) deeper cause (= deficiency)
    - anabolic or catabolic derailment?
    - which hormonal regulator is deficient?
    - which miasma is present?
    - which mineral is deficient?
    - which nutritional group is deficient?
    - which basic psycho-structure is being rejected?
    - which dream symbol corresponds to this?

Step 5: Filling up the deficiency

- What has a counterpolar effect?

the **catabolic effect** (in anabolic disorders) is
- on the psychological level: **living out one's individuality**
- on the metabolic level: **activity up to stress, heat intake**
- on nutritional level: **carbohydrates (especially short-chain)**
- at matrix level: **interference fields, viruses, etc.**

the **anabolic effect** (in catabolic diseases) is
- on the psychological level: **order, schedule, rhythms**
- on the metabolic level: **rest, build-up, movement**
- at nutritional level: **protein, avoidance of carbohydrates**
- on matrix level: **MRT, organ preparations, phytotherapy**
                   tons – especially basic tone
                   sounds vibration, tapping massage

Step 6: Determine hierarchy

What has priority?

Psychic level:
Psychotherapy
Coloroma therapy
Bach flowers
Homeopathy
Psychokinesiology, NLP
Chakra therapy
Meditation, TM
Autogenic training etc.

Metabolic level:
Treatment with SRT, ZMR 703
Coordination of both brain hemispheres
Dietary changes
Adapted exercise
Order therapy, rhythm
Kneipp, massages
Orthomolecular medicine
Ozone, HOT
Light therapy (red light, laser)
Equalizer EQ 103

Matrix level:	MRT 503 (matrix regeneration therapy)
	Permanent stress reduction
	Purification methods
	Tones and sounds (vibration)
	Organ preparations
	Own blood treatment
	Neural therapy
	Acupuncture

Step 7: Control of the healing process
- Accompanying the patient
- Control examinations (metabolism, Luescher test, etc.)

Life-supporting Medicine in practice
The dynamics of a disease process, which is different for each individual patient, is of course very difficult to explain schematically. Therefore, here is another attempt to explain the application of Life-supporting Medicine as vividly as possible. Imagine a new patient coming into the practice who is to be diagnosed and treated with the new knowledge.

Anamnesis
After taking as **comprehensive an anamnesis** as possible, we are particularly interested in the exact circumstances under which the first symptoms appeared and what preceded them. Often special stress situations are reported or infectious diseases that took a gradual course. Here it is also important to find out about previous treatment (suppression or support).

Psychological clarification
The **Coloroma colour test** is suitable for further clarification of the psycho-logical situation. For this, the patient is presented with a colour wheel with the 12 Goethe colours, from which he picks out his favourite colour (without thinking twice) while concentrating on something beautiful. He then decides on a second colour which he dislikes. This time he imagines his symptoms. Additional we use 12 different etheric aromas, which correspond to the characteristics of the colours.

The special thing about this method is the assignment of colours to indivi-dual *characters.* It can be seen immediately which area of life the patient avoids because that is where his conflict potential lays dormant (shadow) and what he/she uses to compensate for this deficiency. (The assignments were found with the collaboration of Prof Max Luescher.)

The result is immediately discussed with the patient in order to immediately set the course for a change in life.

In addition, **Psychokinesiology** can be very helpful. By testing **Bach flowers**, hidden problems of the psyche can also be identified. The psychic correlate of the **extended element teachings** according to B. Koehler is also very informative.

Luescher test

The Luescher test is very important. Here we get much more differentiated statements. The choice of colour is needed for the classification in the **cube of life** according to Luescher/Koehler (cf. Fig. 15 page 69) and enables immediate *access to the deeper cause*.

Expansion of consciousness

Such methods are suitable to find out very quickly well-founded background information about the psycho-energetics of the illness. The results are incorporated into the patient discussions.

The developmental process of the patient, which should lead to an underlying meaning through the *transcendence* of the illness and an *expansion of consciousness* initiated by this, is thus guided along certain concrete paths.

Metabolic state

Right at the first patient contact, a **metabolic measurement** is carried out. This can be done very quickly using bioenergetic methods, and the **stimulus-response behaviour** is also examined immediately in order to find out the **regulatory capacity**. This can be done with the ZMR 703. device.

Also the latest generation of metabolism testing from MedTronik, the MORA*nova* measures automatically and balances immediately afterwards. The SRT is integrated in the VEGA Expert with similar functions.

The therapist can do a lot with this information because it also sets the course for **nutritional recommendations** and all other therapeutic measures.

The determination of the current metabolic situation in connection with the Luescher test alone is sufficient to make fundamental statements about the true, underlying cause (the deficiency). Furthermore, it becomes apparent in which way this deficit is compensated by the patient (cf. Fig. 15).

The metabolism is always tested organ-related, because the *total* metabolism only reflects the sum of all organs, i.e. it is not representative for the disease, but for the remaining health potential. Although this is not uninteresting, it should only be understood as a reference for the recovery process. If possible, the underlying cause is always treated.

The "Luescher Life Cube" thus provides us with clear information about which metabolic situation is primarily responsible for the symptoms and at the same time indicates the actual underlying metabolic derailment.

The Luescher Cube

If we assume that we have a pain patient in front of us in whom the metabolic measurement shows a value of +75° anabolic locally in the area of illness, then we are not at the cause, but only at the place of compensation of a deeper lying disturbance. In the Luescher test, for example, the columns would have shown that blue is rejected (- - 1), but green is preferred (++2). This means that behind the anabolic pain symptoms there is a catabolic metabolic derailment elsewhere (!), accompanied by a lack of HGH. This already points to malnutrition (too many carbohydrates) and at the same time to a water and salt deficiency.

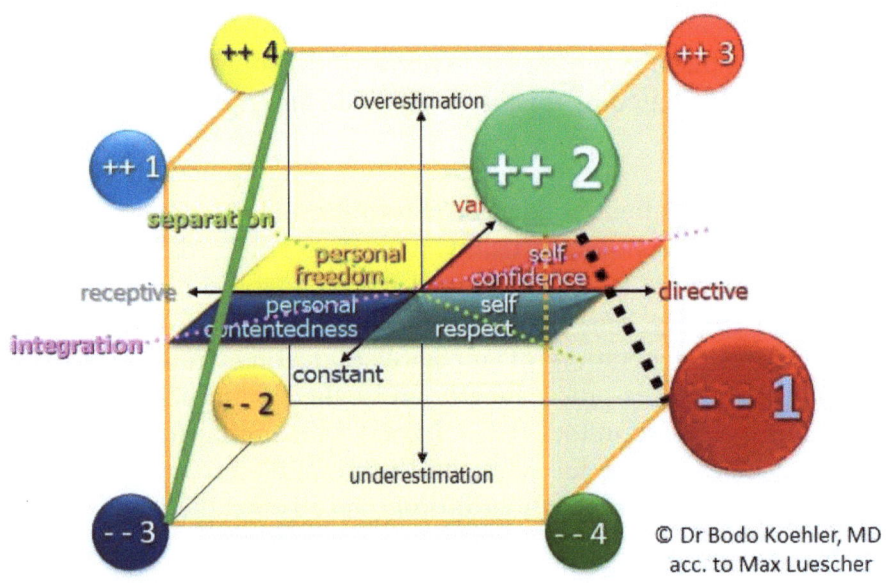

© Dr Bodo Koehler, MD
acc. to Max Luescher

Legend:

■ ■ ■ ■ ■ = actual psycho regulation
━━━━━━ = therapeutic approach

This has very lasting consequences. With this constellation (a high anabolic value compensates for a pronounced catabolic metabolic state), a cancer disease must also be expected, which is why further clarification must take place here. (The pain could be consistent with a paraneoplastic syndrome.) However, the diagnosis can be made in stages (first tumour markers, sonography, etc. before proceeding invasively).

In the Luescher test, the patient chooses green as his preferred colour (++2) and rejects blue (- -1). The predominant symptomatology (acute pain states) is anabolic (+75°). This leads to the following evaluation:

As **compensation** is lived
- Tendency to arrogance
- Excess of anabolic peptides (prevents catabolic compensation)
- Magnesium surplus
- Too much protein is consumed

The **underlying cause** is
- personal discontentedness
- rejection of rest and recovery
- deficiency of growth hormone HGH
- chronic catabolic disorder
- salt deficiency
- water deficiency

Rules of conduct
Especially with this patient, the 10 points of the treatment of civilisation diseases (see page 116) are discussed in any case, as well as the start of a 6-week vegan (!) diet, increased intake of high-quality salt (e.g. Himalaya), in connection with good living drinking water. After that, everything can be eaten again, but with a considerably different emphasis, i.e. more balance, in favour of a complete diet.

Matrix
Also by means of bioenergetic test procedures (e.g. VEGA-CHECK, VEGA-Expert, DFM, EAV, BFD etc.) the **stresses of the matrix** are now determined. First, an overview measurement is made to determine the energy distribution, regulatory disturbances and focal stresses.
With regard to the individual stresses, the heavy metals should be considered first and foremost, taking into account the status of the teeth, whether amalgam fillings are still in there, which act as an obstacle to

therapy. Furthermore, all environmental conditions (geopathy, electro-smog) as well as occupational environmental toxins should be investigated. Vaccination damage can also play a major role and/or extreme eating habits (10 cups of coffee/day or similar).

Physical examination
The oral inspection alone can already tell a lot about the important head foci (tonsils, sinuses, teeth). Peripheral foci (appendix, gall bladder, etc.) as well as scars are revealed by the full body examination. Every knocking pain points to a chronic event.

Hierarchy
After all findings are available, a **hierarchy** is established, which is very helpful in separating the essential from the unessential.
We always treat only the most urgent, as we often then see an improvement in the other disorders. In this context, therapy methods that work with synergistic components and can therefore be used economically are very helpful.

Therapy
Ideally, the matrix can be freed from its stresses with a combination of cupping (suction massage), direct current (reversal of polarity for regeneration) and information therapy (stimulation of the immune system) with the **Matrix Regeneration Therapy (MRT 503).** The treatment takes place 1x per week.

Individual burdens such as heavy metals can be actively tackled by the immune system through phagocytosis, whereby phytotherapy and orthomolecular preparations have a supporting effect. However, this requires a targeted **attention signal**, either by means of nosodes or in a very direct way via Living Systems Information Therapy (LSIT, e.g. with above-mentioned MRT 503, ZMR 703, Equalizer EQ 103, Vegaselect, MORA, BICOM etc.).

In order to increase the **degree of order** in the tissue, which is urgent, sound therapy (also in combination with colours) is particularly suitable, e.g. as basic tone therapy or interval sound therapy, in the form of directly perceptible vibrations in the tissue.
The basis of the **connective tissue**, of which we are made up of more than 80%, is formed by silica, which is increasingly needed during healing processses. It is contained in larger quantities in millet, but can also be supplied in powder or gel form (KlinSiMag® or Sikapur).

In addition to cholesterol and lecithin, the **membrane structure** of the cells consists of lipoproteins (fat-protein compounds). For regeneration, these are needed to a greater extent, which should be done daily with the oil-protein diet according to J. Budwig.

Too little attention is paid in therapy to the formation of new blood vessels. This can be sustainably promoted by flavanals (not to be confused with flavonoids), which are mainly contained in the red peanut shells that make up OPC according to Prof Masquelier.

For the function of the **respiratory chain**, the unsaturated fats, especially linolenic acid, are essential, but also Vit.C and co-enzyme Q 10. Both should be supplied in high doses, whereby the dosage of Q 10 should be chosen according to body weight from 1 to 6 mg/kg bw (e.g. Sanomit Q 10).

Another indispensable part of the therapy are **enzymes,** which are also used in the appropriate dosage (e.g. Phyto-Enzyme 3 x 5 tgl.). However, there are also completely natural forms on the market as fruit extracts, e.g. Noni juice.

Never should the **actual source of energy** be forgotten – the **sun**. In order for the rays emitted by it (braked neutrinos) to be stored as photons by the π-electron clouds of the fats, exposure must logically take place. This means dosed direct sunlight, but without sunscreen, or at least laser or red light.

The **metabolic state** is measured again and again in between, which results in a progression and a statement about the progress of the therapy can be made. The metabolic situation is corrected each time with the metabolic device (VEGA-SRT, ZMR 703, MORA*nova*). This is done on the focus of the disease itself or on the most disturbed meridian (with affixed programmed magnetic strip). This is both a diagnostic and therapeutic procedure that intervenes directly at the level of the regulators.

If it is not possible to dissolve the rigidity, it is essential to clarify the functionning of the endocrine glands (thyroid, adrenal) and possibly substitute them!

A special variant of metabolic therapy consists of forcing the affected, reaction-rigid organ into an anabolic phase (shock phase according to Selye) by means of intensive tapping (several minutes), in order to counteract catabolism with the metabolic device on the third day. This is an elegant way to dissolve many a rigidity. The procedure can be repeated exactly one week later until self-regulation functions stably.

At this point, I would like to remind you once again of the special healing procedure **AM-Integ**, which sustainably promotes the integration of separated tissue sections (inflammation up to tumour).

Parallel to the treatment, the **patient talks**, which are oriented towards the *psychological correlate* that has been worked out, whereby the denied needs of the soul are in the foreground here. Hypericum, magnesium, melatonin, Bach flowers, etc. can be used as support.

The **motivation** of the patients is very important here, as quite a few experience a gain in illness (attention etc.) and therefore hold on to it in the subconscious. The new BEING, which should be achieved in full health, must therefore be more attractive and worthwhile. However, the patient should not "fight" for this, because this means violence and releases aggression, but *let the healing process happen*. However, this can only succeed if the patient does his homework and consistently pursues conflict resolution through forgiving and forgiveness. He should try to reintegrate himself into the cosmic order in order to find his individual centre. It is important to focus on *strengthening his health potential* and to mentally *let go* of the illness.

Insula-amygdala therapy with the Equalizer EQ 103 is particularly suitable for this purpose. Not only does it synchronize the two hemispheres of the brain, but it can also resolve imbalances in stress processing, especially when anxiety is the primary issue. At the same time, vagus stimulation takes place, which can compensate for sympathetic tone.

Balancing therapy *with the Equalizer EQ 103* stands out from all other bioenergetic methods because it unlocks the resources necessary for the healing process by compensating for local deficits in life information. This is made possible by the integrated analog memory.

Control of the healing process
The subjective complaints expressed by the patient should gradually disappear, whereby a time reversal is often noticeable here, i.e. the symptoms disappear in the reverse order in which they appeared. It is quite desirable that earlier, already forgotten problem areas also make themselves known again, in the sense of a final healing reaction.
Even if one day the patient is free of symptoms, the "objective" control examinations should not be neglected. A tumour can continue to grow even though the patient feels well.

The best overview is obtained by accompanying metabolic checks. The repeated Luescher test provides certainty as to whether a fundamental process of consciousness has actually taken place.

Blood tests and imaging procedures can be helpful in individual cases, but their significance should not be overestimated, as they do not allow any statement about the function of an organ.

Whether individual therapy measures restore functionality can be read directly from the metabolic regulation. Only the measurement of the metabolic state creates the necessary therapeutic certainty.

All measures of Life-supporting Medicine have only one purpose: to support the life processes and to transform all elements that are hostile to life, on all levels of being.

Details of this and the necessary practical exercises are taught in seminars. These are either organised by the "International Medical Society for Biophysical Information Therapy (BIT) e.V." in D-Freiburg (www.bit-org.de), or they take place within the framework of congresses such as the Medical Week in Baden-Baden, annually at the end of October.

As already mentioned, the basics can be read in much more detail in the author's book "UNITED life-supporting MEDICINE" (English language), or viewed on the video recordings of a total of 9 seminars on the subject (German language). Reference via www.SoluMed.eu or directly in the www.bod.de/buchshop.

****

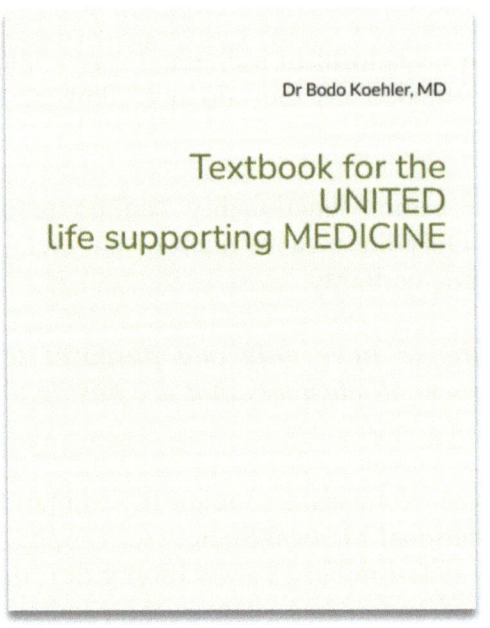

Dr Bodo Koehler, MD

Textbook for the
UNITED
life supporting MEDICINE

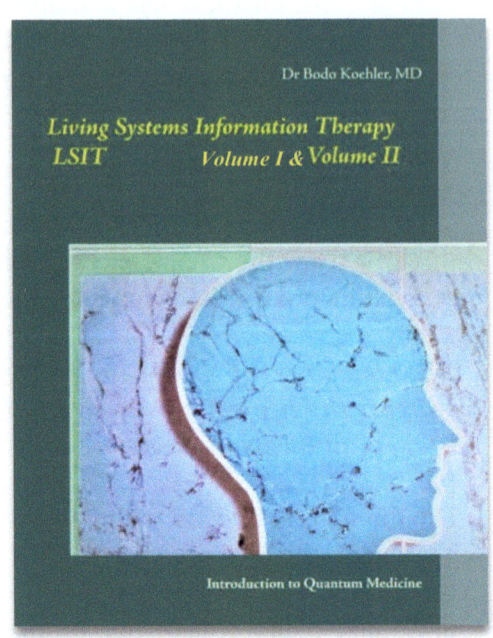

Dr Bodo Koehler, MD

Living Systems Information Therapy
LSIT   Volume I & Volume II

Introduction to Quantum Medicine

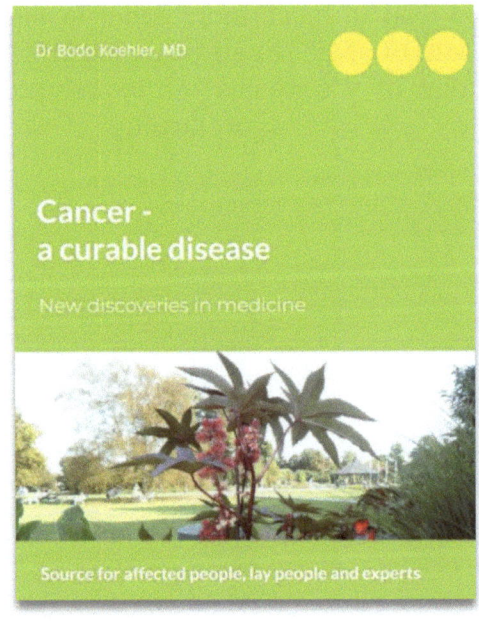

Dr Bodo Koehler, MD

Cancer -
a curable disease

New discoveries in medicine

Source for affected people, lay people and experts

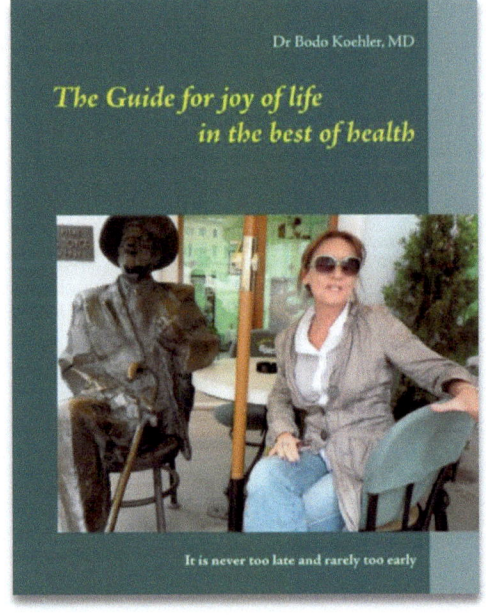

Dr Bodo Koehler, MD

The Guide for joy of life
in the best of health

It is never too late and rarely too early

9.   References

Anemueller, H.,
Ries, J. K.:   "Instructions for a metabolically active diet".
Becker, O.:   "Spark of life", Scherz-Verlag Munich
Berger, L.:   "Music, Magic & Medicine", Junfermann-Verlag 1997
Bischoff, M.:   "Biophotons - the Light in our Cells", V. 2001
Budwig, J.:   "Oil-Protein Diet"
                        "The elementary function of respiration..."
                        "The Death of the Tumour" Vol. 2
Egli, R.:   "The LOLA principle", Editions d'Olt, CH-Oetwil
Egli, R. & F.:   "Illusion or Reality?" Editions d'Olt, CH-Oetwil
Heine, H.:   "Textbook of the Biologic Medicine", Hippokrates-V.
Kaucher, E.:   "Present and Future of Mankind - New Thinking".
Kiene, H.:   "Complem. Medicine – Orthodox Medicine", 1996
Koehler, B.:   "Living Systems Information Therapy", BoD 2020
                        "Cancer – a curable Disease" BoD 2021
                        "Textbook of Symmetropathy", Eigen-Verlag
                        "Textbook of UNITED life-supporting MEDICINE" BoD
                        "Cancer – a curable disease", BoD 2021
Koenig, M.   "The Primordial Word – The Physics of God"
Kriele, A.:   "As in heaven, so on Earth" ch-falk-Verlag 2000
Krueger, W.:   "The Needle's Eye of Colours and Tones",Atom-Harmonik-
Luescher, M.:   "The Law of Harmony in Us", Econ-Verlag Munich
                        "The 4 Colours Man", Goldmann-Verlag 1990
Matheis, R.:   "Leadership Revolution", Verlag Frankfurter Allg.
Meyl/v.Butlar, J.: "Neutrinopower", Argo-Verlag 2000
Meyl, K.:   "Potential Vortex" Volumes I and II, Indel-Verlag VS 90
Peitgen, H et al.: "Chaos – Building Blocks of Order", Springer 1994
Pischinger, A.:   "The System of Basic Regulation", Haug-Verlag
Plichta, P.:   "God's Secret Formula", Langen Müller-Verlag 99
                         "Neutrino or the logarithm of the number zero"
Prigogine,
I./Stengers, I.:   "Dialogue with Nature", Ex Libris Zurich
Rapoport, S.M.:   "Medical Biochemistry".
Schole, J./Lutz: "Regulatory Diseases", BoD
Temelie, B.:   "Nutrition according to the 5 elements", Joy-Verlag 2001
Zabel, W.:   "Nutrition and Cancer", lecture at ZÄN-Congress
Zycha, H.:   "Organon of Wholeness", Haug-Verlag Heidelberg 1996

Notes

Notes

FSC
www.fsc.org

MIX
Papier aus verantwortungsvollen Quellen
Paper from responsible sources
FSC® C105338